D1760282

Homeopathic Prescribing Pocket Companion

Homeopathic Prescribing Pocket Companion

Steven B Kayne

PhD, MBA, LLM, MSc, DAgVetPharm, FRPharmS,
FCPP, FIPharmM, FFHom, MPS(NZ), FNZCP
Honorary Consultant Pharmacist, Glasgow
Homeopathic Hospital, Glasgow, UK
Honorary Lecturer, University of Strathclyde School
of Pharmacy, Glasgow, UK

Lee R Kayne

PhD, MRPharmS, MFHom(Pharm)
Community Pharmacist, Glasgow, UK
Pharmacy Dean, Faculty of Homeopathy, Luton, UK

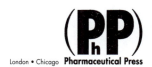

London • Chicago **Pharmaceutical Press**

Published by the Pharmaceutical Press
An imprint of RPS Publishing

1 Lambeth High Street, London SE1 7JN, UK
100 South Atkinson Road, Suite 200, Grayslake, IL 60030-7820, USA

© Pharmaceutical Press 2007

(P.P) is a trade mark of RPS Publishing

RPS Publishing is the publishing organisation of the Royal Pharmaceutical
Society of Great Britain

First published 2007

Typeset by Aptara, New Delhi, India
Printed in Great Britain by William Clowes Ltd, Beccles, Suffolk

ISBN 978 0 85369 6971

A catalogue record for this book is available from the British Library

Contents

Contents

Preface

The idea of this book crystallised in our minds high over Siberia on a flight to Japan in 2005 and the outline was sketched out on the back of a napkin. We both agreed that the time was right to provide practical assistance to colleagues wishing to add homeopathy to their existing skills. With the advent of the modern team approach to healthcare delivery and the granting of prescribing rights to a wider range of health professionals in the UK, the demand for a more comprehensive healthcare service has increased. Minor ailment services, and supplementary and independent prescribing, all provide opportunities to prescribe homeopathic medicines. The over-the-counter (OTC) demand remains buoyant and registered veterinary homeopathic medicines are now available. Despite increasing debate over the use of homeopathic medicines in the NHS, six out of ten Scottish GP practices were prescribing homeopathic or herbal remedies to patients. Research carried out at Aberdeen University has revealed that, out of more than 300 practices surveyed, 49% had prescribed homeopathic treatments and 32% prescribed herbal treatments over the course of a year.[1]

It is acknowledged that there must be some theoretical knowledge underpinning practice and the first part of the book provides a brief introduction to homeopathy and the related disciplines of anthroposophy, biochemic salts and flower therapies. However, we do include in this prescribing guide a review of the evidence supporting the use of homeopathy. It is accepted that, like much of complementary and alternative medicine, homeopathy suffers from a paucity of robust scientific evidence to support its use although many case study reports are available. In Part 2 we aim to assist colleagues in choosing the appropriate homeopathic medicine to treat a range of conditions for which advice is commonly sought, by providing a system of decision tree prescribing flowcharts based on abbreviated drug pictures and supported by supplementary information. In many instances we go beyond simply offering advice on the standard list of polychrest medicines and include lesser known, but none-the-less very useful, medicines.

There will undoubtedly be traditionalists who will feel that this approach cuts too many corners and will dismiss it with contempt. We make no pretence that it could be considered as 'classical homeopathy', or that the charts are totally comprehensive. However, our collective experience over nearly 40 years has shown that homeopathy can be very effective if used in a pragmatic manner, provided that the prescribing is confined to carefully chosen medicines for a range of acute conditions, examples of which are presented.

Unlike orthodox medicine, the homeopathic armamentarium has not increased markedly in modern times, but different approaches to prescribing have developed. Although our writing will inevitably reflect the fact that we are both community pharmacists practising in Scotland, we hope that this book will be of use to colleagues in other professions working in other healthcare environments around the world.

We will be delighted to receive comments and suggestions on this book.

S B Kayne (Steven.Kayne@nhs.net)

L R Kayne (Lee.Kayne@nhs.net)

Glasgow, May 2007

1. Ross R, Simpson R, McLay S (2006). Homeopathic and herbal prescribing in Scotland. *Br J Clin Pharmacol* 62: 647–652.

Acknowledgements

We are grateful for the assistance given by Rebecca and Sorelle in assembling some of the material and to Dr Jay Borneman, Dr Peter Fisher and Evelyn Liddell for their helpful comments on the manuscript.

About the authors

Steven Kayne has practised as a Community Pharmacist in Glasgow for more than 30 years. He is currently Honorary Consultant Pharmacist at Glasgow Homeopathic Hospital and Honorary Lecturer at the University of Strathclyde. Dr Kayne serves on three UK Government Expert Advisory Bodies – the Advisory Board on the Registration of Homeopathic Products, the Herbal Medicines Advisory Committee and the Veterinary Products Committee. He writes and lectures widely in the UK and overseas on a variety of topics associated with complementary and alternative medicines. He has authored, edited and contributed chapters to ten books.

Lee Kayne graduated from the University of Aston and completed his PhD and postdoctoral studies at Nottingham and Harvard Medical School respectively, before returning to his native Glasgow in 1999. He owns a busy community pharmacy offering a full range of orthodox and complementary services and lectures widely on the integration of complementary medicine into pharmacy practice. Dr Kayne is a visiting researcher in Pharmacy Practice at the University of Strathclyde and the current Pharmacy Dean of the UK Faculty of Homeopathy.

PART

1

1

Introduction to homeopathic theory

Complementary and alternative medicine

Complementary and alternative medicine, as defined by the US National Center for Complementary and Alternative Medicine (NCCAM), is a group of diverse medical and healthcare systems, practices and products that are not presently considered to be part of conventional medicine. These systems of medicine are all characterised by the fact that they involve holistic practice – that is, the procedures are individualised according to each patient's circumstances. This means that medicines (or procedures) appropriate for one patient might be totally inappropriate for another – even though the symptoms may be similar. Conversely, the same medicine may be used to treat very different conditions in different patients.

A distinction can be made between complementary and alternative **therapies**, which include those manipulative interventions that generally rely on procedures alone (for example, chiropractic and reflexology), and complementary and alternative **medicine** (for example, aromatherapy, herbalism and homeopathy), which is associated with the use of medicines (or 'remedies' as they are often called). However, the terms are often used interchangeably, as in this book.

The definition of homeopathy

Homeopathy is a complementary and alternative therapy the use of which is based on the **Law of Similars** and involves the administration of ultra-dilute medicines prepared according to methods specified in the various official national homeopathic pharmacopoeias (see Chapter 2), with the aim of stimulating the body's capacity to heal itself.

The status of homeopathy in the UK

In the UK, homeopathy has been available under the country's National Health Service (NHS) since its inception in 1947–48. However, it is not the UK's most popular complementary and alternative therapy by total market value, and it is possible that herbal and perhaps aromatherapy products will be fully reimbursable under the NHS in the foreseeable future. The practice of homeopathy has changed little in the last 200 years or so in the way its medicines have been used. In direct contrast to orthodox medicine, relatively few new medicines have joined the modern homeopath's armamentarium in recent years.

The history of homeopathy

Christian Friedrich Samuel Hahnemann was born just before midnight on 10 April 1755 in Meissen, the ancient town renowned for its porcelain and situated on the banks of the River Elbe, about 100 miles south of Berlin. He qualified as a physician at the Frederick Alexander University in Erlangen in 1779. In 1790, Hahnemann translated and annotated a materia medica written by the eminent Scottish physician William Cullen (1710–90). Hahnemann disagreed with Cullen's suggestion that the mechanism of action of **cinchona bark** in the treatment of **marsh fever (malaria)** was due to its astringent properties. Because he knew of the existence of several astringents more powerful than cinchona that were not effective in marsh fever, he decided to test the drug by taking relatively large doses himself. He found that the resulting toxic effects were very similar to the symptoms experienced by patients suffering from the disease. Hahnemann then tried a number of other active substances on himself, his family and volunteers to obtain evidence to substantiate his findings. In each case he found that the medicines could bring on the symptoms of the diseases for which they were being used as a treatment. Thus he systematically built up considerable circumstantial evidence for the existence of a **Law of Similars** (see below) based on the concept of 'like to treat like'. He called the systematic procedure of testing substances on healthy human beings, in order to elucidate the symptoms reflecting the use of the medicine, a '**proving**'.

In 1810 Hahnemann published his most famous work, the **Organon of the Rational Art of Healing** (commonly simply referred to as '**The Organon**').[1] A total of five editions appeared during Hahnemann's lifetime; the manuscript for a sixth edition was not published for many years after his death. The subject matter in the sixth edition was set out in 291 numbered sections or **aphorisms**, usually denoted in the literature by the symbol § and the relevant section number.

The principles of homeopathy

There are four important principles associated with the practice of homeopathy:

1. **Like cures like**. Hahnemann believed that, in order to cure disease, one must seek medicines that can excite similar symptoms in the healthy human body. This idea is summarised in the Latin phrase *similia similibus curentur*, often translated as 'let like be treated with like'. Thus a medicine such as Coffea tosta, made from toasted coffee beans, might be used to treat insomnia.

2. **Minimal dose**. When Hahnemann carried out his original work he gave substantial doses of medicine to his patients, in keeping with contemporary practice. This often resulted in major toxic reactions; fatalities were not uncommon. He experimented to try to dilute out the unwanted toxicity, while at the same time maintaining a therapeutic effect. Hahnemann found that, as the medicines were serially diluted, with vigorous shaking at each stage, they appeared to become more potent therapeutically. To reflect this effect he called the process **potentisation**. The potentisation process is described in detail below.

3. **Single medicine**. Hahnemann believed that one should use a single medicine to treat a condition. Provings in all materia medicas relate to single medicines and there is no way of knowing whether or how individual medicine drug pictures are modified by combination with other ingredients. In later life Hahnemann did use mixtures of two or three medicines, and there are a limited number of such mixtures still used today, including Arsen iod, Gelsemium and Eupatorium perf (AGE for colds and flu), and Aconite, Belladonna and Chamomilla (ABC for teething). There is a growing tendency for the major manufacturers to combine mixtures of medicines and potencies in one product. These are known as complexes (see Chapter 3).

4. **Whole patient**. The holistic approach to treatment, in which all aspects of a patient's wellbeing are considered, not just local symptoms in isolation (see below).

Treating with homeopathy

Treating with homeopathy involves the following stages:

- Collecting information.
- Matching symptoms reported by a patient with the drug pictures of appropriate medicines.
- Confirming the choice with questions based on modalities (what makes the symptoms better or worse).
- Choosing the correct dose and frequency.
- Following up.

The process is explained in detail in Chapter 4.

Mechanisms of action of homeopathy

The mechanisms of action of homeopathy are not fully understood. Homeopaths consider disease to be an expression of the **vital force** of each individual. Because all individuals are quite different in their expression of the vital force, patients are treated according to their idiosyncratic, rather than their common, symptoms. The symptoms are important only in that they act as an indicator for the selection of an appropriate medicine.

It is believed that the vital force operates on three different levels:

1. General, where changes in understanding and consciousness are recorded (e.g. confusion and lack of concentration) and changes in emotional states are recorded (e.g. anxiety, envy, fear, irritability, love, sadness). These observations serve to build up a picture of the patient's wellbeing.
2. Physical, where changes to the body's organs and systems are recorded (e.g. organ malfunctions and disease).
3. Local, where changes occurring in the immediate vicinity of the patient's problem are considered.

Under normal conditions, the vital force is thought to be responsible for the orderly and harmonious running of the body, and for coordinating the body's defences against disease. However, if the force becomes disturbed by factors such as emotional stress, poor diet, environmental conditions or certain inappropriate allopathic drugs, then illness results. Homeopathic practitioners consider the body's functions to be a melange of all these levels when determining which homeopathic medicine is appropriate to restore the vital force to its 'normal' level.

As stated above, homeopaths look at the **totality of symptoms** rather than at individual aspects of disease in isolation. However, this comprehensive approach is not the only way homeopathic medicines can be used. It is possible to administer medicines chosen for their local effect, in which case the drug picture is reduced to a few highly significant indications (known as 'keynotes') for matching. This approach is used especially for first aid and the treatment of many simple self-limiting acute situations.

Hering's law – the direction of cure

Hering's law, attributed to Dr Constantine Hering (often called the father of American homeopathy), gives an indication of the order in which a condition may be expected to resolve during homeopathic treatment. It states that cure takes place:

- from top to bottom of the body
- from the inside to the outside
- from the most important organs to the least important
- in reverse order of onset of symptoms.

Hence mental symptoms (emotions) might be expected to improve before physical symptoms are resolved, and recent symptoms will subside before longstanding chronic symptoms. A good example of this law in practice is the resolution of asthma, a condition that is often associated with a skin condition. It is not uncommon to see the physical symptoms of asthma improving only to find an underlying skin condition becoming more pronounced.

Proving a drug

Most homeopathic medicines have a **drug picture**, a written survey of the symptoms noted when the drug was given to healthy volunteers, a process known as 'proving the drug'. Hahnemann defined very precise guidelines for carrying out provings. Theoretically, the proving of a substance refers to all the symptoms induced by the substance in healthy people according to Hahnemann's original instructions. Provings are still carried out today, to verify earlier work and to bring new medicines to the homeopath's armamentarium.[2]

Drug pictures

Drug pictures may also contain symptoms derived from the following sources:[3]

- Observations of toxicological effects arising from therapeutic, deliberate or accidental administration.
- Observations of pathological symptoms regularly cured by the medicine in clinical practice. This is the source of many seemingly strange symptoms noticeable in some drug pictures.

In some instances the whole drug picture may be derived from toxicological or clinical observations and not from a true proving at all.

In this book we have used the most important features of various drug pictures to construct prescribing charts that guide colleagues towards the most appropriate medicine for a given condition.

Materia medica and repertories

The drug pictures are collected together in large weighty books called materia medicas and repertories, many of which have been computerised. The former list all the drugs with their drug pictures; the latter list conditions with an indication of the medicines that might be useful in treating them. Within this list there is a hierarchy of type styles in the text to reflect the relative importance of the items mentioned.

The process of choosing a medicine to treat a particular condition by matching symptoms to a drug picture is known as **repertorisation**. A number of such texts are given in Appendix 1.

References

1. Hahnemann C S (1810). *Organon of the Rational Art of Healing*. Dresden: Arnold.
2. Riley D (1996). Homeopathic drug provings: symptom selection criteria and protocol guidelines. *J Am Inst Homeopathy* 89: 206–210.
3. Belon P (1995). Provings. Concept and methodology. *Br Homeopath J* 84: 213–217.

2

Homeopathic medicines

The homeopathic pharmacopoeias

Homeopathic medicines are prepared in accordance with the methods described in various official national homeopathic pharmacopoeias. These have been adopted by the relevant regulatory authorities in the countries concerned. In the EU, the German and French pharmacopoeias are considered to be 'official'. In the USA, the *Homeopathic Pharmacopeia of the US* (HPUS) is the standard. The British homeopathic pharmacopoeia (the latest edition of which appeared in 1999) is not considered to have this status in European law and for many years British manufacturers have relied on the German homeopathic pharmacopoeia (GHP, or HAB in the German abbreviation), with its various supplements, and the French and US pharmacopoeias, for most of their information, particularly with regard to the analysis of starting materials.

The European homeopathic pharmacopoeia that has been in preparation for many years will assume major importance as the number of monographs increases.

It should be noted that some methods of preparing medicines differ between the various pharmacopoeias. There is currently no requirement for manufacturers to state on the label which pharmacopoeial standard their product conforms to. It might be prudent to enquire, especially if a supplier is changed.

The source materials

The source materials used in homeopathic medicines can be classified as follows:

- **Plant material**. Approximately 70% of all homeopathic medicines are prepared from extracts of plant materials and, for this reason, many people confuse homeopathy with herbalism. However, the manner of producing the two types of medicines is quite different. Herbal products are generally the result of an aqueous or alcoholic extraction alone, whereas homeopathy involves an additional dilution process. Either the whole plant may be used or only selected parts, as specified in the pharmacopoeia monographs. Medicines to treat allergies and made from materials such as grass and tree pollens, and moulds, are known as **allergodes** (see Chapter 3).

- **Zoological material**. Examples of medicines derived from healthy zoological material are those derived from the bee and the cockroach. Material from bacterial cultures and healthy animal secretions may also be used. They are generally known as **sarcodes**. Examples include snake and spider venoms, musk oil (Moschus), and secretions of the cuttlefish (Sepia). Musk is obtained from the African civet, a fox-like animal kept in battery accommodation mainly in Ethiopia. Animal fur, hair and feathers may also be used to prepare allergodes, while pathological material yields **nosodes** and may include pus, bodily fluids and diseased tissue (see Chapter 3). Auto-isopathics are similar to nosodes, but are prepared from an individual infected patient's own products (e. g. blood, pustules, urine, warts, verrucae), or from milk from a cow or sheep suffering from mastitis.
- **Chemical material**. Highly purified chemical material is rarely used in the preparation of medicines. Thus, calcium carbonate is obtained from the interspaces of oyster shells and sulphur is obtained from a naturally occurring geothermal source. Chemical material and orthodox drugs may also be used to prepare homeopathic medicines known as **tautodes** (see Chapter 3).

In the USA, terminology differs from the above. The US homeopathic pharmacopoeia provides the following definitions:

- **Isodes**, sometimes called **detoxodes**, are homeopathic dilutions of botanical, zoological or chemical substances, including drugs and excipients, that have been ingested or otherwise absorbed by the body and are believed to have produced a disease or disorder.
- **Nosodes** are homeopathic attenuations of pathological organs or tissues; causative agents such as bacteria, fungi, ova, parasites, virus particles and yeast; disease products; excretions or secretions.
- **Sarcodes** are homeopathic attenuations of wholesome organs, tissues or metabolic factors obtained from healthy specimens.
- **Allersode** is the term used to describe homeopathic dilutions of antigens, i.e. substances that, under suitable conditions, can induce the formation of antibodies. Antigens include toxins, ferments, precipitinogens, agglutinogens, opsonogens, lysogens, venins, agglutinins, complements, opsonins, amboceptors, precipitins and most native proteins.

The preparation of homeopathic medicines

A summary of the manufacturing process is shown in Figure 2.1. It comprises three stages, described below.

Figure 2.1 Summary of the manufacturing process.

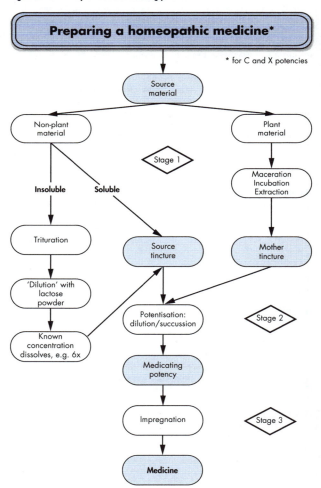

STAGE ONE Preparation of starting materials

Vegetable material

Mother tinctures are liquid preparations resulting from the extraction of suitable vegetable source material, usually with alcohol/water mixtures. They form the starting point for the production of most homeopathic medicines, although some are used orally (e.g. Crataegus) or topically (e.g. Arnica). If a mother tincture is prescribed, the abbreviation Ø is often used. However, the letter Q is also sometimes used – care should be taken to distinguish between the mother tincture and an LM potency (see below). The resulting extract solutions contain on average one part drug to three parts mother tincture, although this strength can vary depending on the species, type of extraction process and the particular pharmacopoeia being used. The resultant solutions are strained to remove any extraneous pieces of debris.

Insoluble material

Chemicals such as Aurum (gold), Graphites (graphite), Silicea (silica) and Sulphur are triturated with lactose in a pestle and mortar. The resulting triturate may be compressed directly into trituration tablets or administered as a powder. More usually, however, trituration continues until the particle size has been reduced sufficiently to facilitate the preparation of a solution ('source tincture' in Figure 2.1), usually achieved after three to six serial dilutions, depending on the scale being used. From this point the standard potentisation procedure described below can be followed.

Soluble chemicals

In the case of soluble chemicals, solutions of known concentration in distilled water or alcohol can be initially prepared as the starting solution. This is called the 'source tincture' in Figure 2.1.

STAGE TWO Potentisation (also called dynamisation or attenuation)

With the exceptions noted above, most mother tinctures are serially diluted in a special process that increases the homeopathic strength (although the chemical concentration decreases), for which reason the process is known as **potentisation**.

The solution resulting from admixture of the two liquids at each dilution is subjected to a vigorous shaking with impact, known as **succussion**. The number of times the vials should be shaken is not specified in the pharmacopoeia and may, depending on the manufacturer, be anything from 10 to 100 or more, but within each manufacturing process it remains constant. Succussion is still carried out by hand in some pharmacies, but some large-scale manufacturers have mechanical shakers.

There are several different methods of dilution, of which the **Hahnemannian** method is the most widely used (Figure 2.2).

Figure 2.2 The potentiation process (Hahnemannian).

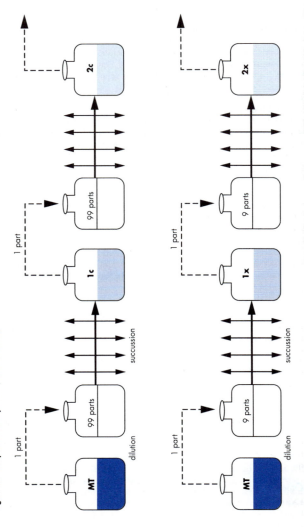

MT, mother tincture

Table 2.1   Centesimal potencies

Centesimal potency	Concentration	Dilution
1 (1c or 1cH)	10^{-2}	1:100
6 (6c or 6cH)	10^{-12}	$1:10^{12}$
12 (12c or 12cH)	10^{-24}	$1:10^{24}$
30 (30c or 30cH)	10^{-60}	$1:10^{60}$
200 (200c or 200ch)	10^{-400}	$1:10^{400}$
M*	10^{-2000}	$1:10^{2000}$
10M*	$10^{-20\,000}$	$1:10^{20\,000}$

*Korsakovian dilutions.

Table 2.2   Decimal potencies

Decimal potency	Concentration	Dilution
1x (D1)	10^{-1}	1:10
6x (D6)	10^{-6}	$1:10^{6}$
12x (D12)	10^{-12}	$1:10^{12}$
30x (D30)	10^{-30}	$1:10^{30}$

In the Hahnemannian **centesimal method** of potentisation, one drop of mother tincture is added to 99 drops of triple distilled alcohol and water diluent in a new, clean, screw-cap glass vial. After the initial process, successive serial dilutions are made, accompanied by succussion, using fresh glass vials at each stage until the solution reaches 3c, 6c, 12c, 30c, 200c and so on; the number refers to the number of successive 1 in 100 dilutions and 'c' indicates the centesimal method. The suffix may also be expressed as 'cH' or may be omitted entirely, leaving just the number. The stages are summarised in Table 2.1

In the **decimal scale**, one drop of mother tincture is added to nine drops of diluent. This is indicated in the UK by a number and the letter 'x' (e.g. 6x), although in other countries the scale may be indicated by 'dh' after the number (e.g. 6dh) or by 'D' before the number (e.g. D6).

At the higher centesimal dilutions letters are sometimes used alone. Thus the 1000 dilution level is 1M or simply M, 10 000 is XM or 10M and 100 000 is CM (Table 2.2). These high potencies are usually made using the much quicker Korsakovian method (see below), but use the same notation.

Other potentisation methods

LM (or Q) potencies are triturated to the third centesimal level with lactose before being diluted according to a 1 in 50 000 scale (Figure 2.3). LM potencies are sometimes referred to as 'Q' potencies, which can often be confused with a mother tincture. However, an LM will always have a number

Figure 2.3 Medicating process for LM potencies.

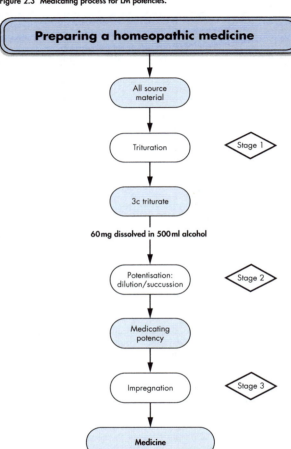

Preparing a homeopathic medicine

All source material

Trituration — Stage 1

3c triturate

60 mg dissolved in 500 ml alcohol

Potentisation: dilution/succussion — Stage 2

Medicating potency

Impregnation — Stage 3

Medicine

to designate the potency level, e.g. LM1 or Q1, LM6 or Q6, whereas a mother tincture will simply use the letter alone. Homeopaths often instruct patients to succuss liquid LM potencies before taking each dose.

In the **Korsakovian** method, medicines are prepared by adding a measured volume of mother tincture to an appropriate volume of diluent and the resulting solution succussed thoroughly (Figure 2.4). Liquid is then removed from the vial by suction or inversion, leaving droplets of solution adhering to the container wall. New solvent is then added, the vial agitated

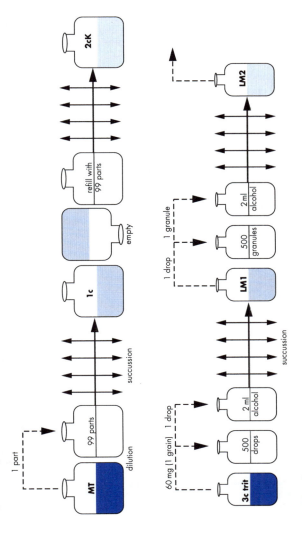

Figure 2.4 The potentisation process (Korsakovian and LM).

MT, mother tincture

vigorously and the process repeated. Korsakovian potencies are usually denoted by a number showing the number of serial dilutions, followed by the letter 'K' (e.g. 30K). This method and K potencies are rarely used in the UK, certainly at low potencies. However, as stated above, this method is often used in the case of very high potencies, which may not realistically be made by the Hahnemannian method. Thus, a 1000 potency may be referred to as 1M, M (as above) or even MK.

Mechanisms of potentisation

One of the fundamental tenets of homeopathy is the concept of potentisation, and yet it continues to be one of the major stumbling blocks to its widespread acceptance, with many sceptics claiming that it is just a myth.[1] It is not known how Hahnemann came upon the procedure of potentisation, but it probably arose from his knowledge of chemistry and alchemy. Geometric and dynamic models have been constructed to try and explain how medicines can be therapeutically active at such extreme dilutions.[2] There is some evidence to indicate that the structure of solvent molecules may be electrochemically changed by succussion, enabling them to acquire an ability to 'memorise' an imprint of the original medicine. It is acknowledged that this concept is difficult for many highly trained personnel with scientific backgrounds to accept. The simplest suggestion is that succussion may merely facilitate a complete mixing.

STAGE THREE Presentation

Dose forms

Solid dose forms

In orthodox medicine, tablets and capsules are made in different forms to control the speed at which the active ingredient is delivered. This is not necessary in homeopathy, so the choice of 'carrier' is governed by convenience rather than therapeutic efficiency. Common solid dose forms are illustrated in Figure 2.5.

- **Tablets** are about 100 mg in weight and are similar to the classic, biconvex, plain white product used widely in conventional medicine. They are manufactured commercially from lactose and appropriate excipients. On an industrial scale, blank lactose tablets, or indeed any of the solid dosage forms, can be surface inoculated by spraying on the medicine in an alcoholic tincture or as a syrup in a revolving pan, rather like the old method of sugar coating. The exact amount of medicine to be applied to ensure an even covering is validated using dyes. On a small scale in the pharmacy, the solid dose forms may be placed in glass vials and medicated by placing drops of liquid potency in strong alcohol on the surface, the number of drops used depending on the amount of solid dose form being medicated. The container is agitated in a manner similar to succussion, to disperse the medicine throughout the dose form.

Figure 2.5 Solid dose forms.

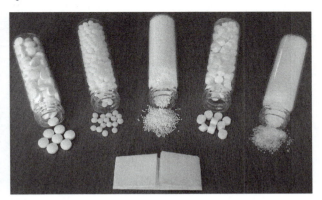

- **Individual powders** are made from lactose impregnated with medicating liquid potency and are useful where small numbers of doses are required.
- **Pills and granules** are small spheres, usually sucrose, which resemble cake decorations. The former are approximately 3–4 mm in diameter, while the latter are very tiny, approximately 0.9 mm in diameter and often referred to as 'poppy seeds'.
- **Crystals** are sucrose, and have the appearance of granulated sugar.
- **Soft tablets** are loosely compressed lactose tablets that melt in the mouth.

Liquid dose forms
- **Mother tinctures** may be given orally (e.g. Crataegus, Valerian), usually in water. They are often applied topically (see below).
- **Liquid potencies** are serial dilutions made from mother tinctures but in a lower concentration of alcohol (typically 20–30%) than that used to medicate solid dose forms (typically 95%). They are usually given in water but the drops may be placed directly on the tongue, or on a sugar cube.
- **Injections** There are a number of injectables on the market, of which the most widely prescribed in the UK are variants of Mistletoe used in the management of cancer, e.g. Adnoba (Abvoba Heilmittel Gmbh, Pforzheim, Germany) and Iscador (Weleda).

Topical dose forms
- **Mother tinctures** may be applied topically, either singly (e.g. Arnica for bruising, Thuja for warts or Tamus for chilblains) or in mixtures (e.g. Hypericum and Calendula – widely known as 'Hypercal').
- **Ointments, creams, gels, lotions, liniments** (generic and patent) and **oils** contain between 5 and 10% of mother tincture, or in a few cases where no mother tincture exists liquid potency (e.g. Graphites,

Sulphur), incorporated in a suitable vehicle. Available topical preparations include Arnica (bruising), Calendula and Hypericum (superficial wounds), Rhus tox/Ruta (sprains and strains), Tamus (chilblains), and Thuja (warts and verrucae).

- **Eye drops** have caused manufacturers licensing difficulties and at the time of writing are restricted to prescription on a named patient basis in the UK. Argent nit, Calendula, Cineraria and particularly Euphrasia eye drops are all extremely useful and are likely to prove very popular should they become more widely available.

The containers

There has been much discussion as to whether plastic or glass containers are appropriate for solid dose forms. The traditionalists still favour neutral glass containers, suggesting that there is a possibility of chemicals leaching into the plastic. Little work has been done to investigate whether the fears of those eschewing plastic have a firm foundation. There have also been suggestions that the glass may play some part in 'holding' the potency. Again, these have not been substantiated.

Liquids are packed in glass dropper bottles. The major suppliers use amber screw cap bottles with a plug in the neck, with a channel that facilitates the delivery of one measured drop (0.05 ml). Silicone rubber teat droppers are rarely used as again there is some concern over leaching.

Legal classification of homeopathic medicines

Manufactured homeopathic medicines are subject to careful scrutiny to ensure that they are of the highest quality and safety. In the UK they have been treated as medicines since the inception of the NHS in 1948 and are available on medical prescription just as orthodox medicines are. As a result, they are subject to rules governing their manufacture and supply.

Human use

In Europe, there are three routes by which homeopathic medicines can be registered:

1. Products with limited claims of efficacy based on bibliographic evidence, and injections, may be registered under UK national rules.
2. Products that are 4x and above may be registered on the basis of quality and safety only (i.e. making no claims of efficacy) under an abbreviated European scheme.
3. Full registration with substantiated claims of efficacy as for orthodox medicines supported by clinical trials. No homeopathic medicine has been registered under this classification.

Registered homeopathic medicines for human use may be sold in the UK without restriction in a wide range of retail outlets. Exceptions include certain formulations such as eye drops and injections that may contain un-licensed ingredients and are restricted to medical prescriptions on a named patient basis. Some unlicensed medicines obtained from homeopathic manufacturers holding special manufacturing licences may be classified as pharmacy only (P) and should not be placed on open shelves. Homeopathic medicines may be prepared extemporaneously by pharmacists in a registered pharmacy if they have appropriate expertise.

In the USA, homeopathic medicines are subject to the Food, Drug, and Cosmetic Act of 1938 and regulations issued by the Food and Drug Administration (FDA).[3] Pre-market approval is by way of monograph approval by the Homeopathic Pharmacopoeia Convention of the United States (HPCUS).[4] While homeopathic drugs are also subject to the FDA's non-prescription drug review, the FDA has not yet used this authority. However, manufacturing, labelling, marketing and sales of homeopathic medicines are subject to FDA compliance rules. These rules, with the exception of provisions for expiration dating, tablet imprinting and finished product testing, are functionally identical to the rules for their allopathic counterparts. Good manufacturing practice standards for homeopathic and allopathic drugs are the same. Subject to the relevant FDA regulations, homeopathic medicine indications may be given on the label and there are no limitations on where homeopathic medicines can be sold.

Veterinary use

The normal UK category is Authorised Veterinary Medicine – General Sales List (AVM-GSL). If a registered homeopathic veterinary product exists then it must be supplied even if it is requested generically.

A vet may use medicines 'off-label' under the 'prescribing cascade', subject to a strict hierarchy. These provisions apply to both orthodox and homeopathic practice.

- If there is no licensed veterinary medicine available for a particular condition or for use in a particular species, similar veterinary products may be used.
- If there are no suitable veterinary products, a human medicine may be prescribed.
- If no suitable human product is available, a pharmacist or a vet may prepare the required medicine extemporaneously provided that they have the necessary expertise.

The position with respect to the over-the-counter (OTC) supply of homeopathic veterinary products was under review at the time of writing, pending clarification of the European position. Under a grandfather clause in the 2006 Veterinary Regulations, products that were on the market in the UK prior to 1996 may be registered with the Veterinary Medicines Directorate (VMD) and placed on the market without further action. Nosodes and sarcodes do not qualify for grandfather rights.

References
1. Isbell W, Kayne S B (1997). Potentization – just a myth? *Br Homeopath J* 86: 156–160.
2. Schulte J (1999). Effects of potentisation in aqueous solutions. *Br Homeopath J* 88: 155–160.
3. Borneman J P, Field R L (2006). Regulation of homeopathic products. *Am J Health-Syst Pharm* 63: 86–91.
4. Food, Drug, and Cosmetic Act of 1938, Pub. L. 103–417, 52 Sta. 1041 (1938), as amended and codified in 21 U. S. C. §321(g)(1) (1938).

3

Types of homeopathic medicines, practitioners and practices

Types of homeopathic medicines

Homeopathic medicines are often classified according to how they are used in practice.

Classical medicines

Most homeopathic medicines fall into this group. They are used according to Hahnemann's original method of matching up the patient's symptoms to the drug picture. A period of consultation lasting up to an hour or more may be necessary to obtain sufficient information for the practitioner to prescribe on the basis of the 'totality of symptoms' rather than simply on local symptoms. This effectively reduces the number of conditions that may normally be treated in most community pharmacies to minor ailments and simple self-limiting conditions.

Constitutional medicines

In any given population the following may be observed:

- People react to homeopathic medicines with different levels of intensity.
- Some people respond especially well to a particular medicine; among people in this unique group, certain physical and mental characteristics appear to be common (e. g. skin texture, hair colour, height and weight). Further, these people also tend to suffer from similar complaints; for example, Pulsatilla and Sepia are both used for pre-menstrual tension. However, 'Pulsatilla ladies' tend to be weepy while 'Sepia ladies' tend to be tall and slim with a darker complexion.
- Parallels can often be drawn between certain characteristics shared by people in this group, and the physical or chemical properties of a medicine. Pulsatilla (the windflower) is a slender flower that bends in

the wind, a characteristic that may be considered as being analogous to having a changeable temperament. However, it must be stressed that homeopathy does not generally function like the 'Doctrine of Signatures' popularised by herbalists in the seventeenth century. In simple terms, this doctrine was the idea that God marked everything He created with a sign or signature that indicated the purpose of the item's creation and where it might be used therapeutically.

The constitutional characteristics of the patient prevail in the absence of disease. They are also aspects of the individual that may intensify during illness to become symptoms. Particular physical characteristics, body functions and psychological traits may become exaggerated.

If a person's constitutional medicine coincides with the symptom picture being presented, there is a strong possibility of a favourable outcome.

The use of constitutional medicines is a skill that eludes most novice prescribers. Prescribers need to know a great deal about the patient and the medicine, and the use of constitutional medicines is not recommended unless appropriate knowledge and experience have been gained.

Polychrests

This group of 20 to 30 medicines, examples of which are listed in the box below, are extremely important in practice. They form the basis of most commercially available homeopathic ranges, because they lend themselves to prescribing based on abbreviated drug pictures without protracted consultations. Over-the-counter (OTC) prescribing in pharmacies is generally,

Examples of medicines considered to be polychrests	
Aconite	Ignatia
Apis mell	Ipecac
Argent nit	Kali bich
Arnica	Lycopodium
Arsen alb	Merc sol
Belladonna	Nat mur
Bryonia	Nux vom
Calc carb	Pulsatilla
Carbo veg	Rhus tox
Euphrasia	Ruta grav
Gelsemium	Sepia
Graphites	Silica
Hepar sulph	Sulphur
Hypericum	Thuja

but not exclusively, based on polychrests. Although they are used mainly for first aid and acute situations in the OTC environment, polychrests have drug pictures that show a very wide spectrum of activity affecting many body tissues and are often indicated in chronic disease and constitutional prescribing.

Isopathic medicines

An explanation of the different groups of isopathic medicines and terminology used in Europe and the USA is provided in Chapter 2. Most isopathic medicines are administered on the basis of the principle *Aequalia aequalibus curentur* – 'let same be treated by same' – rather than the classical 'let like be treated by like'. Most have not been subjected to provings and therefore do not appear in standard texts, although some do appear in the materia medica by Julian.[1]

Allergodes

Allergodes can be used effectively provided that the patient knows the source of the allergy or skin testing results are available. There are geographic variations that may need to be considered (e. g. for pollens, trees or moulds). Allergodes can be effective in the treatment of a range of allergic reactions (see Chart 3, Allergies).

Nosodes

There are various childhood illnesses represented among the nosodes, including whooping cough (pertussin) and German measles (rubella). There are also tropical nosodes like cholera and malaria sometimes claimed to be 'vaccines' (see box below). Some historical nosodes have drug pictures, although their use is limited to rather specialised circumstances. Examples include Influenzinum, Bacillinum (see Chart 14, Cold and flu) and Psorinum (see Chart 22, Eczema and dermatitis).

Sarcodes

Many of these medicines (particularly those derived from snake and spider venoms) have comprehensive drug pictures and may be used following repertorisation in the normal manner.

Nosodes and sarcodes as 'vaccines'

The word 'vaccine' is sometimes used erroneously to describe nosodes and sarcodes that are given both prophylactically and as a treatment, with the aim of stimulating the auto-immune response against a disease. It should be noted that none of these medicines is a true vaccine and there is little evidence that they can confer any protection against a disease when given prophylactically. It is appropriate to exert some voluntary control when certain nosodes are being used. The UK Faculty of Homeopathy counsels against the use of any medicines by members of the public in such circumstances (see http://www.trusthomeopathy.org).

Tautodes

Tautodes (also known as tautopathic medicines) are used for the isopathic treatment of adverse drug reactions, allergies and chemical irritation thought to be directly caused by the source material chosen. Very few of the tautodes have drug pictures. Examples include commercial vaccines and drugs.

Complex medicines

The mixing of different medicines and different potencies in one container, selected for their combined effect on particular diseased states, is known as 'complex' prescribing. This is very popular in France and Germany, where it is not uncommon to have 15–20 medicines ranging from very low to high potencies in the same preparation, with indications for use on the label. It is likely that many of these complex mixtures will appear on the UK market within the foreseeable future (see page 29).

Other types of related medicines

Anthroposophical medicines

A related form of homeopathy is known as **anthroposophy**. Although the nature of anthroposophical medicines is essentially the same as homeopathic medicines, there are some important differences in the manufacturing process. Great care is taken in collecting raw materials for preparing anthroposophical medicines. Vegetable material is grown using methods of biodynamic farming, a development of organic practice where the soil is fed to improve its structure and fertility. Soil additives are restricted to homeopathic medicines only; all other hormones and chemicals are excluded. Due cognisance is taken of the natural cycles of the moon, sun and seasons. The first growth of plants is harvested and composted, and a second crop grown on the composted material. The process is repeated, and the third generation of plants is used to prepare the medicine. Manufacturers prefer to produce their own source material whenever possible. Anthroposophical pharmacies use different temperatures during the manufacturing process, according to the particular medicine involved. Aconite, said to exhibit the properties of 'coolness', is prepared at a lower temperature than Crataegus, a medicine acting on heart muscle and therefore active at body temperature. Paying attention to the temperature during preparation can be seen as helping to relate the medicines to human use. The medicines are extracted, diluted and used without potentisation, or prepared using the homeopathic process of serial dilution and succussion.

Homotoxicology

This was the brainchild of German doctor Hans-Heinrich Reckeweg (1905–85), and is also based on homeopathy. Drawing on a vast knowledge of herbal lore and medicines, Dr Reckeweg compounded a store of remedies that combined folk medicine and basic plant pharmacology. Homotoxicologists endeavour to identify and treat the underlying toxic causes of ill health, rather than merely to suppress symptoms. The therapy is used widely in Germany but is less well known in the rest of the world.

The biochemic tissue salts

The tissue salts are often included under the homeopathic umbrella, although their inventor insisted that they were quite separate from homeopathy.

Dr Wilhelm Heinrich Schüssler, a German homeopathic physician from Oldenburg, introduced a number of inorganic substances in low potency to his practice in 1872, and developed the idea of biochemic tissue salts.

Proponents cite unhealthy eating practices that could lead to deficiencies of various salts considered to be vital for healthy functioning of the body. It is argued that this situation may be corrected by taking tissue salts.

There are 12 single biochemic tissue salt medicines, together with some 18 different combinations. They are made by a process of trituration, each salt being ground down with lactose sequentially up to the sixth decimal potency (6x) level. The resulting triturate is then compressed directly into a soft tablet. Although most of the salts are soluble, there is no intermediate liquid stage, and surface inoculation is not used as it is thought to render the tissue salts ineffective. The tablet readily dissolves in the mouth, releasing fine particles of mineral material that can be absorbed into the bloodstream through the mucosa.

The salts are often referred to by a number from 1 to 12 in order of their names. They are listed in the box below.

The biochemic tissue salts*
1. Calc fluor (calcium fluoride)
2. Calc phos (calcium phosphate)
3. Calc sulph (calcium sulphate)
4. Ferrum phos (iron phosphate)
5. Kali mur (potassium chloride)
6. Kali phos (potassium phosphate)
7. Kali sulph (potassium sulphate)
8. Mag phos (magnesium phosphate)
9. Nat mur (sodium chloride)
10. Nat phos (sodium phosphate)
11. Nat sulph (sodium sulphate)
12. Silicea (silica)

*Used in the 6x potency, usually as soft tablets

For many ailments, more than one tissue salt is required. In order to simplify treatment there are a number of combination medicines containing three, four or five different salts, usually referred to by the letters A to S and given specific indications. Two examples are:

- Combination A contains Ferr phos, Kali phos and Mag phos and is used for sciatica and neuralgia.
- Combination S contains Kali mur, Nat phos and Nat sulph and is used for stomach upsets.

Flower remedies

This group of medicines is not homeopathic but is included in this book because they are often used in conjunction with homeopathy (see Chart 4, Anxiety and shock). They fall somewhere between homeopathy and herbalism and are not currently subject to legal classification in the UK. Flower remedy therapy treats predominantly mental and emotional manifestations of disease, relying on the administration of remedies derived from the flowering parts of plants.

There are many variants of flower remedies, but the original and best known are the Bach flower remedies popularised by the immunologist Edward Bach. In 1934 Dr Bach established a healing centre in a small house at Mount Vernon, Oxfordshire, UK, where many of the plants used in his remedies could be grown or were available as wild specimens in the immediate area. He subsequently completed his collection with a further 26 remedies, and considered the final total of 38 to be sufficient to treat the most common negative moods that afflict the human race.

These 38 remedies can be split into six groups according to their principal use:

- Fear (aspen, cherry plum, mimulus, red chestnut, rock rose).
- Uncertainty (cerato, gentian, gorse, hornbeam, scleranthus, wild oat).
- Insufficient interest in present circumstances (chestnut, clematis, heather, honeysuckle, impatiens, mustard, olive, water violet, white chestnut, wild rose).
- Oversensitivity to influences and ideas (agrimony, centaury, holly, walnut).
- Despondency or despair (crab apple, elm, larch, oak, pine, star of Bethlehem, sweet chestnut, willow).
- Overcare for the welfare of others (beech, chicory, vervain, vine, rock water).

One of the difficulties of using Bach remedies is that, during the resolution of disease, mental symptoms are likely to change, requiring the administration of different treatments. In order to deal with this there is an extremely useful combination of five Bach flower remedies, known as **five-flower remedy** or **Rescue Remedy** (see Chart 4, Anxiety and shock). It was so named for its stabilising and calming effect on the emotions during a crisis. The remedy comprises cherry plum (for the fear of not being able to cope mentally), clematis (for unconsciousness or the 'detached' sensations that often accompany trauma), impatiens (for impatience and agitation), rock rose (for terror) and star of Bethlehem (for the after-effects of shock). This remedy is often used in place of Arnica, where the mental symptoms resulting from a traumatic episode or overwork are more evident than the physical. Bach rescue cream is a skin salve that is claimed to help a wide range of skin conditions. The cream contains the same five remedies as the Rescue Remedy drops, plus crab apple (for a sense of uncleanliness). It is broadly used for conditions similar to those for which Arnica might be applicable. However, it is difficult to understand how topical use in this way fits in with the concept of treating mental symptoms.

The practice of blending flower remedies appears to be growing. One recently launched range includes nine combination remedies with names such as 'male essence', 'bowel essence' and 'night essence'.

Administration

Frequency of administration depends to a large extent on each individual patient. If the mood is transient then only one dose might be appropriate, while, if the condition persists, repeated dosing could be appropriate.

Patients should be instructed to add 2–4 drops of the Bach flower remedy to a cold drink of their choice (fruit juice or still mineral water are both acceptable) and the mixture sipped every 3–5 minutes for acute problems until the feelings have subsided. The liquid should be held in the mouth for a moment before swallowing. If no suitable beverage is available, 4 drops of the remedy may be placed under the tongue. For longer use a dose should be taken four times daily.

Homeopathic practitioners

In the UK, Ireland and many other English-speaking countries, most health professionals have responded reactively to a demand for homeopathy from clients, rather than encouraging its use proactively, although with improved access to training this position is changing. In these countries homeopathy may be practised not only by statutorily registered qualified health professionals, but under common law, also by professional (i.e. non-medically qualified) homeopaths and by lay homeopaths with no formal training. A professional homeopath is a practitioner who has qualified from a recognised college of homeopathy, and practises in such a way that all the criteria for registration requested by their professional body continue to be fulfilled. Most suitably trained health professionals, and some professional homeopaths, are able to use homeopathy under the NHS in the UK.

Common law permits freedom of choice of the patient to choose the healthcare provisions that they feel appropriate, and the freedom of people to practise homeopathy if they so wish. The main drawback of such a liberal system is that it allows a person to set up as a homeopath with little or no training, although this situation is likely to change with new controls brought in following the Shipman case.

Registered healthcare professionals practising homeopathy and professional homeopaths have quite separate educational facilities and voluntary governing bodies. Practice by the former may be supervised by the Faculty of Homeopathy (http://www.trusthomeopathy.org/faculty). The Faculty was founded in 1950 by act of Parliament. Joining the Faculty is voluntary; the body has no statutory powers and there appears to be no imminent decision by the UK government to require homeopaths to be statutorily registered. The Faculty accredits training courses for health professionals, awarding the qualifications of Licentiate (LFHom with appropriate suffix) as a basic qualification for all health professionals, Diplomate (DFHom) as an intermediate qualification (currently available only to dentists, pharmacists and podiatrists), and Full Membership (MFHom) and Fellowship (FFHom) for the medical, nursing, pharmacy and veterinary professions. The postgraduate courses in medical homeopathy are claimed to be the fastest growing of any speciality and currently more than 300 doctors hold the MFHom qualification. In addition there are 350 with the LFHom and an unspecified number of prescribers occasionally prescribing homeopathy who do not have a formal qualification.

Professional homeopaths registered with the Society of Homeopaths in Northampton, UK (http://www.homeopathy-soh.org) may use the letters RSHom (or FSHom) after following a course of instruction and a period of clinical supervision. Another body is the UK Homeopathic Medical Association (http://www.the-hma.org), whose full members have fulfilled similar requirements. The British Institute of Homeopathy also provides courses. These practitioners use the initials MHMA after their name. Few homeopathic medicines are classified as prescription only medicines (POMs); the majority may be supplied in response to private prescriptions written by professional homeopaths.

Despite their substantial training in well-established colleges, the professional homeopaths were formerly regarded with disdain by medical homeopaths, an opinion that continued into the 1980s. However, discussions are now proceeding on an amicable basis and the two groups are moving together, albeit rather slowly.

There are **NHS homeopathic hospitals** in Bristol, Glasgow, Liverpool, London and Tunbridge Wells (see Appendix 1). There may be other NHS-funded clinics in certain areas. The British Homeopathic Association (http://www.trusthomeopathy.org) can provide further details.

Interestingly, Germany also has two classes of practitioners – doctors (95% of whom practise some form of complementary medicine) and 'Heilpraktikers'. The latter group, literally translated as 'health practitioners', developed in the years before the Second World War, when doctors did not have a monopoly on the delivery of healthcare. At present the ratio of practising 'Heilpraktikers' to physicians is about 1:4. They are not obliged to undertake formal medical training, but are obliged to take a 'test' that is administered by the Local Health Authority. If a candidate fails he or she may continue to resit until successful. The Heilpraktiker's activities are comparable to the British professional homeopath, except that they tend to use several different therapies concurrently, and place more emphasis on diagnostic procedures.[2]

Approaches to the practice of homeopathy

There are many schools of thought around the world as to how homeopathy should be practised with respect to the choice of medicine and potency and frequency with which medicines should be administered. There is no established 'norm'. Writers on homeopathy frequently refer to 'classical' or European homeopathy, usually with the implication that this is the most complete and authoritative version of Hahnemann's views and most closely represents his methods. However, such claims do not correspond with the historical facts. Campbell has criticised the notion that there is a standard or pure form of homeopathic practice and argues instead that the so-called 'classical' homeopathy is really a complex mixture of ideas drawn from a variety of sources.[3]

There are broadly three ways in which homeopathic medicines are administered in Europe and in other countries where European influence is strong (except for France where the approach often differs):

- One medicine at a time in a single dose or repeated doses is prescribed by those claiming to be 'classical' or unicist homeopaths. Generally favoured by homeopaths in the UK, this is said to be the 'classical' approach to homeopathy. However, Hahnemann changed his ideas several times, especially towards the end of his life, and so the term 'classical' could be applied to several different methods of using medicines in various low, high and LM potencies and not just unicist prescribing.
- More than one medicine at a time, given simultaneously in alternation or concurrently. This is called 'pluralist' prescribing and claims to treat more than one aspect of a patient's condition. It is common in France, Germany and Italy, and where medicines from these countries are available.
- Mixtures in one container of different medicines and different potencies, selected and combined for their combined effect on particular diseased states. This method is known as **'complex' prescribing**. Classical homeopaths claim that this is not true homeopathy as there is no individual matching of the symptom and drug picture. They argue that, as no provings have been conducted on the mixtures, there is no homeopathic basis for their use. In practice the evidence of effectiveness for such interventions is mixed. A German non-randomized, observational study demonstrated the effectiveness of treating the upper respiratory symptoms of the common cold,[4] while Jacobs et al. found a combination medicine did not significantly reduce the duration or severity of diarrhoea in a sample of Honduran children.[5]

In this book the prescribing charts featured in Part 2 are designed to lead to a single medicine, but in some circumstances more than one medicine may be appropriate (see Chapter 5).

References

1. Julian O (1979). *A Materia Medica of New Homoeopathic Remedies*. Beaconsfield: Beaconsfield Publishers Ltd.

2. Ernst E (1996). Towards quality in complementary health care: is the German 'Heilpraktiker' a model for complementary practitioners? *Int J Quality Health Care* 8: 187–190.

3. Campbell A (1999). The origins of classical homeopathy? *Comp Ther Med* 7: 76–82.

4. Schmiedel V, Klein P (2006). A complex homeopathic preparation for the symptomatic treatment of upper respiratory infections associated with the common cold: an observational study. *Explore (NY)* 2: 109–114.

5. Jacobs J, Guthrie BL, Montes G A *et al.* (2006). Homeopathic combination remedy in the treatment of acute childhood diarrhea in Honduras. *J Alt Complement Med* 12: 723–732.

4

Prescribing and dispensing homeopathic medicines

Source of a request for a homeopathic medicine

In the UK, the supply of a homeopathic medicine may be in response to:

- an NHS prescription signed by a doctor, dentist or pharmacist with appropriate prescribing rights as a result of a consultation and subject to the conditions of their practice
- a pharmacist's NHS prescription generated through a minor ailments service
- a pharmacist's NHS prescription when acting as a supplementary prescriber as part of a shared care plan
- a pharmacist's verbal prescription following an OTC consultation ('counter prescribing')
- a prescription signed by a veterinary surgeon for a registered veterinary medicine or a human homeopathic medicine under the 'prescribing cascade' (see Chapter 2)
- a prescription from a healthcare professional or a professional homeopath (also known as non-medically qualified practitioner or NMQP)
- an over-the-counter (OTC) request from a client. In this case the stimulus prompting the purchase of a medicine may come from a practitioner who will either issue a formal prescription or give verbal instructions on what to buy. Other purchasers are influenced by friends, family and the media.

Prescribing a homeopathic medicine

The prescribing of homeopathy at the initial stage is no different to orthodox medicines. The major differences are in the selection of the appropriate medicine for each patient (see Part 2).

Figure 4.1 Chart of prescribing procedures.

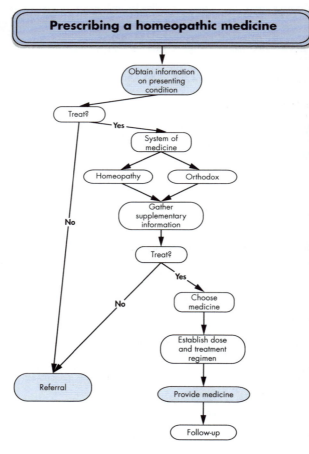

Prescribing a homeopathic medicine

Obtain information on presenting condition

Treat?

Yes

System of medicine

Homeopathy

Orthodox

Gather supplementary information

Treat?

Yes

No

Choose medicine

No

Establish dose and treatment regimen

Referral

Provide medicine

Follow-up

The prescribing process is summarised in Figure 4.1 and comprises the following eight steps:

1. Obtaining basic information on the condition being presented.
2. Taking a decision on whether to treat in the pharmacy or to refer.
3. Taking a decision to treat with homeopathy or orthodox medicine.
4. Gathering supplementary information.
5. Deciding on a particular medicine.
6. Establishing a dose regimen.

7. Providing the medicine.
8. Follow-up.

Step 1: Gathering basic information

The problem of whether to treat or refer is one with which the pharmacist is entirely familiar. In order to take this decision in an informed manner some basic information is required and the questioning process described by the well-known acronym WWHAM (Who is the medicine for? What is the medicine for? How long have the symptoms been present? Action already taken? Medicines currently being taken for other reasons?) may help reinforce the information proactively supplied by the patient.

Step 2: Deciding whether to treat or refer

With experience, and within the bounds of one's competency, the decision to treat or refer may be taken without an in-depth investigation (see Figure 4.1). It will be based on a variety of factors including the severity and type of symptoms being presented, the length of time during which symptoms have been experienced and the patient's health status.

Step 3: Deciding on homeopathy or orthodox medicine

Having decided to treat, the next question is whether to treat with homeopathic or allopathic (orthodox) methods. The patient might express a strong wish to be treated by homeopathy or there may be no suitable OTC allopathic product available. For example, requests for help with examination nerves can be effectively met with Argent nit or Lycopodium, and Nux vom may be suggested with confidence to women suffering from nausea during the first trimester of pregnancy.

The prescribing charts included in the second part of this book will assist in identifying the most appropriate medicine. Homeopathy might also be indicated for patients with an existing extensive portfolio of medication where adding extra drugs might cause worries about interactions.

Homeopathy may not be appropriate in all situations – for example, where the body is suffering a substantial deficiency or imbalance or there is major infection present it will be necessary to deal with the cause of the problem directly as well as treat the symptoms on a local level.

Step 4: Gathering supplementary information

Before one can choose an appropriate medicine to counter prescribe, information must be gained from:

- The patient – signs and symptoms, both observed and reported.
- The practitioner's observational and listening skills.
- The practitioner's own knowledge and limits of competency.
- The prescribing charts (see Part 2) and/or other resources.

A useful acronym to use when assessing a case is provided by the letters **LOAD**, standing for **L**isten, **O**bserve, **A**sk and **D**ecide.

- **LISTEN** to what the patient tells you about his or her symptoms.
- **OBSERVE** the patient's general demeanour, appearance, temperament, etc.
- **ASK** the patient appropriate questions to learn more about the condition.
- **DECIDE** what to do next, after assessing the information provided.

Given the restrictions on resources in most pharmacies it is not possible to pursue extended consultations. This means that the conditions being treated are likely to be restricted to simple self-limiting conditions, although some chronic conditions may be tackled as experience grows.

Step 5: Deciding on a particular medicine

If all the preparatory work in step 4 has been carried out assiduously, then choosing the medicine from the appropriate prescribing chart is not as daunting as it might first appear. There is another acronym that might be useful here. **ACT** stands for **A**ssess, **C**onfirm, **T**alk.

- **Assess**. With all the requisite information one can now choose an appropriate medicine using the prescribing charts provided in Part 2 of this book.
- **Confirm**. Having chosen the medicine most likely to be of assistance it is advisable to repeat a few key questions shown in the chart to allow confirmation of the medicine. **Modalities**, where shown, are particularly useful. Examples of modalities are that symptoms are made better or worse by the application of heat or cold to the affected part, by movement and exposure to warm or wet weather or whether they vary with time of day.
- **Talk**. It might also be appropriate to give some general information on homeopathy, especially if you are acting proactively rather than reactively to a request for homeopathic medicines from the client in addition to counselling (see below).

Step 6: Generating a prescription

The following information should be provided to ensure that a prescription is correctly interpreted:

- **Name of medicine**. Care should be taken to ensure that the abbreviations used are correctly interpreted, e. g. Staph. could be Staphylococcinum or Staphisagria. In some cases, full names of medicines will be required, e.g. Mercurius could be Merc sol, Merc viv, Merc cyan, etc. If in doubt, revert back to the practitioner.
- **Potency**. Normally in the UK the potency will be on the centesimal scale (most commonly 6c, 12c, 30c or 200c) or on the decimal scale (most commonly 6x). Very high potencies such as M, 10M, 50M and

CM may also be requested. Some pharmacists believe that high potencies should not be used to self-treat and may restrict their supply to prescription or very small quantities. Mother tinctures may be designated with the abbreviation Ø.

- **Dose form**. The carrier is thought to be insignificant therapeutically (although this has not been proven experimentally) but there may be other reasons why one or other form is preferred. For example, infants or animals may require granules, crystals or powders; patients with an intolerance to lactose may require a sucrose-based dose form or a liquid.
- **Quantity**. Solid dose forms in the UK are often made available in 7 g, 14 g or 25 g glass vials, indicating the capacity of the container. These correspond to approximately 70, 125 and 250 tablets respectively, depending on the physical characteristics of the tablet. Liquid potencies and mother tinctures are usually supplied in 5, 10, 30 and 50 ml bottles that can deliver their contents drop-wise.
- **Dose**. It is preferable to have the dose specified, rather than 'as directed'. Some of the homeopathic dose regimens are complicated and oral instructions easy to forget, especially by older patients. The adult dose is usually two tablets and by convention it is generally stated that the dose for a child under 12 years should be half that of an adult (i.e. one tablet instead of two). The directions for granules are often rather bizarre – 'Take 10–20 granules twice daily' is not uncommon. This does not mean the patient has to physically separate out 10–20 granules but is an indication of how much they should take, i.e. 'a pinch'. In the absence of precise instructions, 'sufficient to cover the cap-liner' might be an appropriate amount, although this obviously depends on the size of the bottle (and therefore cap) used. Liquid medicines are given as drops usually diluted with water, although they may sometimes be taken directly on the tongue. The following dose frequencies are suggested and are summarised in Figure 4.2:
  - **first aid situations:** the medicine may be given frequently – even up to every 10–15 minutes for 6 doses in some cases. Here the term 'first aid' refers to a suggested initial treatment for any condition being treated, not just for an injury as in orthodox medicine. A suitable potency would be 30c.
  - With **acute prescribing** the 30c dose should be taken three times daily for up to 7–10 days, reducing on improvement.
  - In **chronic conditions** frequencies of once or twice a day or less at the 6c potency for 4–6 weeks may be more appropriate. After the timescales indicated the case would normally be reviewed and a decision made on follow-up action (see below).

Step 7: Providing the medicine

Finally, the medicine is dispensed and the patient counselled (see below).

It is often useful to provide a method of recording progress during the course of treatment, particularly if the medicine has been prescribed and/or supplied in the pharmacy. If the patient can see a positive trend it will

Figure 4.2 Chart showing dose options.

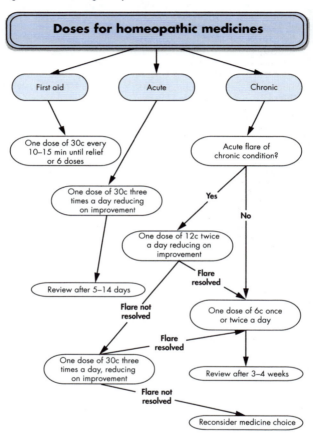

help with concordance as well as giving feedback to the prescriber. A hybrid version of a visual analogue scale and the Glasgow Homeopathic Hospital Outcome scale has been used by pharmacists in the west of Scotland for some years and is illustrated in Figure 4.3. Patients are asked to place a tick in the appropriate box on the grid having assessed their condition using a +4 (cured) to −4 (much worse) scale. The slope of the best-fit line through the ticks gives an indication of outcome trend. This information can be used to help decide the appropriate action at follow-up (see below).

Figure 4.3 Outcome card.

• How my symptoms have changed •

Day	Much worse −4	−3	−2	−1	0	+1	+2	+3	Much better +4	Notes
e.g.			✗							
1										
2										
3										
4										
5										
6										
7										
8										
9										
10										
11										
12										
13										
14										
15										
16										
17										
18										
19										
20										
21										
22										
23										
24										
25										
26										
27										
28										
29										
30										
31										

Step 8: Follow-up

The treatment should be reviewed after the periods stated above. The approach to follow-up is summarised in Figure 4.4:

- The medicine has proved successful and may be discontinued.
- The outcome is not satisfactory, but the patient has not been taking the medication according to instructions. In this case instructions should be given to restart the course of treatment.
- The outcome is unsatisfactory, but the patient has returned too soon. The course should be completed before further action.
- The patient appears to have completed the treatment but the outcome is unsatisfactory. Consider changing the medicine or dose or referring.

Dispensing homeopathic medicines

- **Original pack dispensing**. To avoid contaminating the medicine, especially in the early days of dealing with homeopathic prescriptions,

Figure 4.4 Follow-up chart.

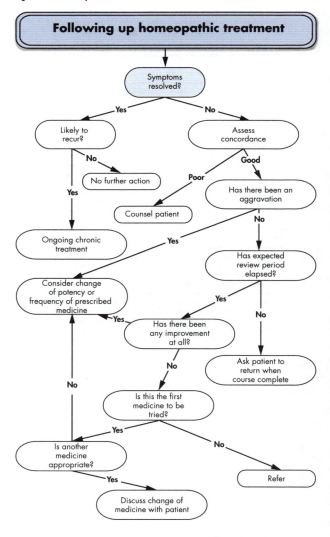

Following up homeopathic treatment

Symptoms resolved?

Yes → Likely to recur?

No → Assess concordance

Likely to recur? — No → No further action

Assess concordance — Poor → Counsel patient

Assess concordance — Good → Has there been an aggravation

Likely to recur? — Yes → Ongoing chronic treatment

Has there been an aggravation — No → Has expected review period elapsed?

Has there been an aggravation — Yes → Consider change of potency or frequency of prescribed medicine

Has expected review period elapsed? — Yes → Has there been any improvement at all?

Has expected review period elapsed? — No → Ask patient to return when course complete

Has there been any improvement at all? — Yes → Consider change of potency or frequency of prescribed medicine

Has there been any improvement at all? — No → Is this the first medicine to be tried?

Is this the first medicine to be tried? — Yes → Is another medicine appropriate?

Is this the first medicine to be tried? — No → Refer

Is another medicine appropriate? — No → Consider change of potency or frequency of prescribed medicine

Is another medicine appropriate? — Yes → Discuss change of medicine with patient

it is probably wise to issue an original pack nearest to the amount specified.

- **Breaking bulk**. If you do decide to break bulk then solid dose forms should not be handled or tablets counted in a tablet counter but transferred by first shaking into the lid. In the case of powders only the precise number of powders prescribed should be issued to the patient. Many suppliers will provide, for example, 1–10 or 11–20 powders at the same cost – it is not good practice to order 10 to fulfil a prescription for 3 powders unless you can guarantee the storage conditions of the 7 powders to be retained in the pharmacy.

- **Extemporaneous dispensing**. It makes commercial sense to license only around 35 homeopathic medicines so many will have to be dispensed extemporaneously. The techniques involved are rather specialised and outwith the scope of this book. For further information the reader is referred to a more comprehensive text.[1]

- **Unlicensed products**. If you do not have the necessary expertise you can obtain extemporaneously prepared homeopathic medicines from manufacturers who have special manufacturing licences. Under these circumstances the homeopathic medicine is considered to be unlicensed and responsibility for safety rests with the prescriber. However this should not cause any anxiety because the chance of an adverse episode is minimal.

- **OTC products on prescription**. There is a range of licensed homeopathic and anthroposophical products available for OTC supply, which may also be supplied on NHS prescription. As with all homeopathic (and orthodox) medicines, pharmacists should be aware of the possibility that these items may be cheaper for the patient to purchase OTC if they are liable to pay prescription charges. OTC products may also be supplied under minor ailment and supplementary prescribing services. You should ensure that the dose form of the product is as prescribed – for example some OTC products may be pills and not tablets, and a 'special' may be requested.

Labelling

Dispensed medicines should be labelled in the normal way and a clear indication given of the name and potency. Occasionally it may be necessary to reinforce complicated instructions with a separate sheet of written instructions. If you have obtained an extemporaneously produced medicine from a Specials Manufacturer it is good practice to include the batch number and expiry date on the label, as shown in Figure 4.5.

Counselling

- **Information on homeopathy**. Most patients will know that they are likely to receive a homeopathic prescription if they attend a suitably qualified practitioner, but some may not. There may be evidence of some anxieties about the validity of the therapy and you may consider it necessary to say a few words about the general features of homeopathy so that the patient is aware of the type of treatment being given. You

Figure 4.5 Labelling of a homeopathic medicine.

Antimonium tart 30c
14g Soft Tablets

Two tablets to be taken three times a day,
reducing on improvement
       BN:123456   Exp: 05/2009
Manufactured by ABC Homeopathic Pharmacy

Mr P. Andham   **1st June 2007**
Friendly Pharmacy, 10 Park Road, Anytown AA10 144
Keep out of the reach of children

---

may say that it is safe, will not interfere with other medicines and is tailored to their particular requirements. It is difficult to give exact guidelines because it depends very much on the person involved. However, you should be ready to say something appropriate. Try to keep your comments concise and unbiased. Remember also to tell the patient not to stop taking any prescribed orthodox medication.

- **Aggravations**. Occasionally, taking a homeopathic medicine may cause an exacerbation of symptoms and it may be prudent to alert the patient to this possibility (see below).
- **How to take the medicine**. The other important information concerns taking the medicine. Because the active ingredient is placed on the surface of the dose form and is absorbed through the oral mucous membranes a number of precautions should be taken:
  - Solid dose forms should not be handled, to prevent deterioration due to bacterial or chemical contamination. They should be transferred to the mouth by way of the container cap (Figure 4.6). If dropped on the floor they should be discarded.
  - Solid dose forms should be allowed to dissolve in the mouth rather than being chewed and/or swallowed.
  - Liquid medicines should be held in the mouth for 20–30 seconds before swallowing.
  - Medicines should be taken half an hour before or after food, drink, tobacco, other medication or sweets. Aromatic flavours are thought to inactivate homeopathic medicines. Ideally peppermint-flavoured toothpaste should be avoided, but, if it is used, the patient should wait at least 30–60 min after cleaning their teeth and the mouth should be rinsed out thoroughly with water before taking the medicine.
  - Medicines should be kept in the original container and stored in a cool dry place.
  - Existing allopathic medication should not be stopped without the permission of the original prescriber.

Figure 4.6 How to take the medicine.

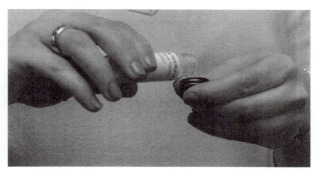

a

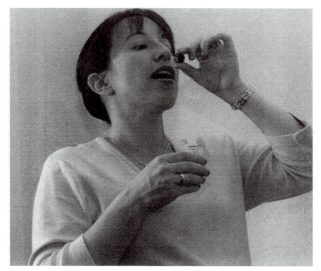

b

Endorsing an NHS prescription

Homeopathic medicines have been available under the UK NHS since its inception in 1948 and the prescription form (or in Scotland, additionally a GP10A a stock order) should be endorsed with the amount supplied and the supplier's name, if not given by the prescriber. Adding the trade price (ex-VAT) and 'ZD' (for the majority of specially ordered medicines) will be helpful to the Prescription Pricing Authority. If in doubt you will find your suppliers very willing to give advice. Increasingly the costs of private homeopathic treatment are being met by health insurance schemes but as the situation is changing from month to month patients should be advised to check with their own insurer before presenting their prescription. In most cases, an insurance scheme will cover the cost of the consultation but not the cost of the medication at the point of supply, and the patient may be surprised to be asked to pay. Issuing a receipt specifying the supply of a homeopathic medicine will usually allow the patient to claim the cost back.

Dispensing of homeopathic veterinary prescriptions

Where there are no licensed veterinary homeopathic veterinary medicines, human homeopathic medicines may be dispensed on veterinary prescriptions under the provisions of the prescribing cascade (see Chapter 2).

Sale of homeopathic medicines OTC

Several ranges of the most popular licensed homeopathic medicines are available for OTC sale. Other items may be made extemporaneously, as noted above.

Safety issues

There is currently no robust system available for collecting information on adverse reactions suspected of being due to homeopathic medicines. The Pharmacy subcommittee of the European Committee on Homeopathy (http://www.homeopathyeurope.org) has piloted a 'yellow card' scheme that uses cards specially adapted for homeopathic use. If an adverse reaction is suspected, all relevant information should be sent to the Medicines and Healthcare products Regulatory Agency (MHRA, http://www.mhra.gov.uk) in the UK or to the WHO Uppsala Monitoring Centre (http://www.who-umc.org).

Potential sources of concern over safety issues include the following.

Inappropriate treatment

Most ranges of homeopathic medicines available commercially for OTC sale are designed to be used for the treatment of simple self-limiting conditions. Some may also be used for ongoing conditions such as back pain or soft tissue injuries. Clients who request unusual medicines or who return repeatedly to purchase the same medicine should be gently reminded that advice from a physician or registered homeopath might be appropriate to confirm that their condition lends itself to self-treatment.

It is vital that all practitioners offer advice and treatment only according to their levels of competency. Patients whose problems fall outwith these boundaries should be referred to suitably qualified colleagues.

Side-effects

Adverse reactions have been investigated using electronic databases, hand searching, searching reference lists, reviewing the bibliographies of trials and other relevant articles, contacting homeopathic pharmaceutical companies and drug regulatory agencies in the UK and the USA, and by communicating with experts in homeopathy.[2] It was concluded that homeopathic medicines in high dilutions, prescribed by trained professionals, were probably safe and unlikely to provoke severe adverse reactions. It is difficult to draw definite conclusions because of the low methodological quality of reports claiming possible adverse effects of homeopathic medicines. Some isolated cases in the literature have also been highlighted by Barnes.[3] From time to time one meets a sensitivity to lactose that can be overcome by using a sucrose-based carrier or a liquid potency.

Aggravation

In about 10% of cases the patient's condition may be exacerbated within 2–5 days of taking a medicine. Typically a skin condition may become worse after taking a low-potency medicine. Such a reaction usually occurs only the first time the medicine is introduced to a treatment. This reaction, known as an **aggravation**, has been described as an adverse drug reaction (ADR) and in the sense that it is unwanted by the patient it might be considered thus. When told of this possibility, many patients will say that 'they do expect to get worse before they get better with this sort of treatment'. Far from being upset by the apparent ADR they consider an aggravation a sign that the medicine is working.

If an aggravation appears, the patient should be instructed to cease taking the medicine until the symptoms subside and then recommence, taking the medicine at a lower frequency. If the symptoms continue to get worse when the medicine has been temporarily suspended, then it is likely that the wrong medicine is being taken. Patients who are receiving prescribed medication should be advised to consult their practitioner because ways of dealing with aggravations can differ.

Interactions

There is no evidence that homeopathic medicines interfere with any concurrent orthodox medicines and indeed they are particularly useful to treat many conditions in people who are taking a large number of orthodox medications. It is thought that steroids may inactivate homeopathic medicines to some extent and, while this potential interaction is certainly not dangerous, it could reduce their expected effectiveness.

Some homeopathic medicines are considered to antidote or inactivate other medicines in some circumstances. Examples of incompatible medicines are shown in Table 4.1.

Aromatherapy products are claimed to inactivate homeopathic medicines and should not be taken during treatment. Traditionally, homeopaths advise patients to refrain from consuming coffee, tea, chocolate and spicy food and using highly flavoured toothpastes when taking homeopathic medication. However, there is little evidence that such abstinence is in fact necessary.

Table 4.1 Examples of incompatible homeopathic medicines	
Homeopathic medicine	Incompatible with
Aconite	Glonoine
Allium cepa	Arnica
Apis mel	Aconite, Carbo veg
Argent nit	Phosphorus, Rhus tox
Aersen alb	Merc sol
Bryonia	Pulsatilla
Calc carb	Hepar sulph
Camphor	All other medicines
Cantharis	Causticum
Colocynth	Coffea, Nux vom
Ignatia	Belladonna, Chamomilla
Kali bich	Lachesis
Nux vom	Cocculus, Coffea
Sepia	Ant tart
Sulphur	Hypericum

From Blasig and Vint.[5]

Evidence supporting use of homeopathy

There is much circumstantial evidence from case studies, from both patients and practitioners, that homeopathy does work. However, robust scientific evidence is sparse – much of the reported research suffers from poor methodology.[4] Examples of the latter include dubious accuracy of test materials, inappropriate measurements and poor randomisation techniques. This is unfortunate to say the least because, increasingly, decisions on whether to use or purchase homeopathic services require evidence of positive outcomes and value for money. None the less there is a wide perception among members of the public that homeopathy can help.

Broadly, homeopathic research falls into six main categories:

1. Randomised controlled placebo studies designed to demonstrate that homeopathy is not merely a placebo response and satisfy criticism from sceptics.
2. Clinical trials to establish efficacy of specific remedies.
3. Physico-chemical studies on mechanisms of action.
4. Audit and case study collection to establish effectiveness and improve the use of homeopathy.

5. Attitudes and awareness studies and sociological research to determine why and how homeopathy is used.
6. Cost-effectiveness studies.

It is beyond the scope of this prescribing companion to discuss the evidence base for homeopathy in detail. The reader is referred to specialist texts on this subject for such information.[1,4,6]

The current position with regard to homeopathy may be summarised as follows.[6] The most enthusiastic proponents of homeopathy would claim that:

- it is totally safe and free from adverse reactions
- it can be used for almost every condition at any time in any patient
- it treats the whole patient as well as the local symptoms of disease.

The true position is rather more circumspect:

- Homeopathy is generally as safe as is claimed and can be used in some situations where orthodox medicine is inappropriate, although more rigorous collection of data on suspected adverse reactions is necessary.
- It cannot be used to resolve the cause of biochemical imbalances or inadequacies (e. g. hormonal imbalance or iron deficiency) but may be useful in reducing associated symptoms.
- More evidence is necessary to support the use of homeopathy in complex conditions and problem and treatment modelling is necessary.
- There is evidence that in some circumstances homeopathy appears to be capable of influencing well-being and local disease.
- There are economic benefits to accrue from using homeopathy.

References

1. Kayne S B (2006). *Homeopathic Pharmacy*, 2nd edn. Edinburgh: Churchill Livingstone.
2. Dantas F, Rampes H(2000). Do homeopathic medicines provoke adverse effects? A systematic review. *Br Homeopath J* 89(suppl 1): S35–38.
3. Barnes J (1998). Complementary medicine: homeopathy. *Pharm J* 260: 492–497.
4. Ernst E, Hahn E G (eds) (1998). *Homeopathy. A critical approach*. Oxford: Butterworth-Heinemann.
5. Blasig T, Vint P (2001). *Remedy Relationships*. Greifenberg: Hahnemann Institute.
6. Dean M E (2004). *The Trials of Homeopathy*. Stuttgart: KVC Verlag, 245–246.

PART

2

5

Introduction to the prescribing charts

This remainder of this book comprises a series of detailed prescribing charts for some of the most common conditions for which patients seek advice. These charts will allow homeopathy to be prescribed with as full a consideration of the symptom picture and modalities as possible, despite the time constraints often experienced in a busy practice.

The presenting condition may be located in the index (entries in italics) and the symptoms traced on the relevant chart to identify the most appropriate medicine to treat the symptoms reported by the patient. Brief notes and a materia medica in tabular format are also given to assist in the choice of treatment. Where experience shows that a **frequently indicated medicine** can be identified, it is given in the notes under the abbreviation **FIM**. It is worth considering this first.

The charts are designed to suggest a single medicine for a condition; however, more than one medicine may appear to be indicated in some cases. Retracing the stages and further careful questioning should clarify the choice. When the medicine has been chosen, confirmatory questions can then be framed using the materia medica tables. These tables include modalities ('Better' and 'Worse' for columns) and other selected features of the drug picture appropriate to the condition being treated. Four reference texts (see below) have been used, together with our own experiences, to achieve a consensus view. It is unlikely that you will obtain an exact match with all the features given, but one or more of the features noted should strike a chord with the patient.

In conditions such as sciatica and cold/flu, patients may present with changing symptoms. Here, it is often beneficial to prescribe more than one medicine. These can be taken in an alternate fashion or, if available, as a specially prepared combination medicine. With changing symptoms, it is also important to establish when it is time to change the medicine(s), or indeed stop a successful treatment. This comes with experience, but generally the medicine dosage may be reduced as soon as improvement is experienced, increasing again only should the symptoms return.

Advice on potency and dosage regimens specific to a condition is given, where applicable, in the notes on the page facing the relevant chart. In the absence of any specific guidance, medicines may be prescribed as shown in Figure 4.2. Note that medicines used initially in a first aid scenario may be continued at a lower acute dose if required for a longer period.

The majority of the medicines recommended in the following charts are polychrests, and will be stocked in most pharmacies offering a homeopathic service. However, as a very individualised system of medicine, there are conditions in which some less well-known medicines or combinations may be required in specific circumstances. A specialist homeopathic manufacturer will be able to prepare and supply these medicines.

Appendix 3 details the various charts on which a given medicine may appear. This will assist in answering the common question, 'What is medicine x for?'. However, it should be noted that many medicines appear in multiple charts, indicated for widely varying conditions. For example, Lycopodium appears in nine charts and is indicated in symptoms ranging from anxiety to ear problems to flatulence. This illustrates how difficult it is to answer the above question satisfactorily, especially as Lycopodium may also be a constitutional medicine and bear little if any relationship to the actual symptoms being experienced (see Chapter 3).

This book has been written principally for healthcare professionals – therefore, while some suggestions have been made for lifestyle advice and concurrent conventional treatments in the notes accompanying each chart, these are by no means exhaustive and are not intended to replace the skill and professional judgement of the practitioner in each individual case. In addition, no glossary of medical terms or list of referral criteria is provided. Standard notation for twice daily (bd) and three times daily (tds) is used.

Reference texts used for the prescribing charts and supplementary information

Boericke W (2005). *Homoeopathic Materia Medica with Repertory*, 2nd British edn, 5th impression. Sittingbourne: Homoeopathic Book Service (various editions available).

Gemmell D (1997). *Everyday Homeopathy*. Beaconsfield: Beaconsfield Publishers.

Murphy R (2000). *Homeopathic Remedy Guide*, 2nd edn. Blacksburg, VA: HANA Press.

Vermeulen F (2000). *Concordant Materia Medica*. Haarlem, NL: Emryss Publishers.

1 Abscesses and boils

- Hypericum/Calendula tincture useful as a mouthwash for abscesses in mouth; may also be used to create a moist dressing – dilute 10 drops in 100 ml boiled/cooled water and use up to qds as required.
- Hypericum/Calendula 5% cream/ointment useful topically.

Homeopathic medicine	Better	Worse	Other
Apis	Open air, uncovering skin	Heat (in bed), touch	Stinging pain and swelling around abscess
Belladonna	Light covering	Heat and touch	Sudden onset, hot
Ferrum phos	Cold application	Touch, and at night	Can be associated with red inflamed eyes
Hepar sulph	Warmth	Cool	Lesions tend to suppurate
Lachesis	Warm application	After sleep	Blue–black swelling around boil
Merc sol	In the morning	Late afternoon	Skin may be cold and clammy
Silica	Warmth	In morning and after washing	Eruptions itchy

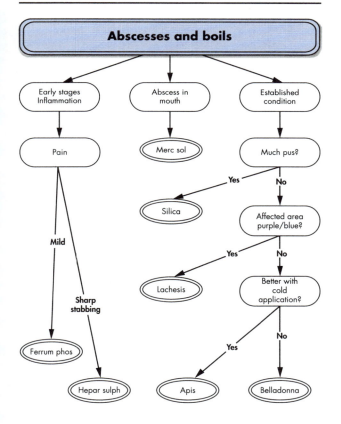

2 Acne

- Topical Calendula 5% cream/ointment useful on individual spots or infected areas.
- Calendula tincture may be applied neat to greasy skin.
- Hypericum/Calendula tincture may be useful on painful lesions – may be applied neat but may sting. If so, dilute 5 drops into 100 ml boiled and cooled water and wash.
- If the most appropriate remedy is not effective after 3–6 weeks, a constitutional medicine may be more suitable – a detailed consultation would be required; consider referral.

Homeopathic medicine	Better	Worse	Other
Belladonna	Light covering	Touch	Skin dry and hot
Gunpowder	Cool	Heat	Bursting headaches possible
Hepar sulph	Warmth	Touch and cool air	Papules prone to suppuration and bleeding. Excessive sweating. Cold sores
Kali brom	After physical activities	Cold weather	Pustules, itching, worse on chest, abdomen and face. Sleep restless
Psorinum	Heat, warm clothing	Cold	Dry skin. Eczema behind ears, crusty eruptions
Rhus tox	Warm, dry weather	During wet weather and at night	Intense itching, red swollen skin
Sanguinaria	Sleep	On the right side and touch. In the spring	Red, blotchy eruptions
Selenium	In evening	In hot weather	Dry, scaly eruptions
Silica	With warmth and in the summer	In cold air. After washing	Pale, waxy skin
Sulphur	Dry, warm weather	Warmth after washing and in morning	Dry, scaly skin
Sulphur iodatum	Cool air and in winter	After exertion and heat	Itching, especially on ears and nose. Cold sores

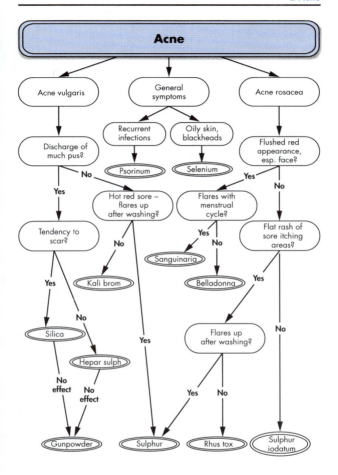

3 Allergies

There are three ways of approaching the treatment of allergies:

1. Advise the patient to avoid the allergen. This may or may not be practical, depending on the lifestyle and whether the allergen has been identified. Simple advice like not allowing a pet to sleep on the bed at night or avoiding certain foods might be appropriate.
2. Choosing a homeopathic medicine on the basis of 'like to treat like' (see Chapter 1 and the dedicated prescribing charts for Hay fever, Itch, and Bites and stings).
3. Using allergodes, isopathic medicines made from the allergen causing the condition. This is based on the principle of 'same to treat same' (see Chapter 1).

Topical Urtica cream may provide an option if the patient presents with an urticarial type of rash.

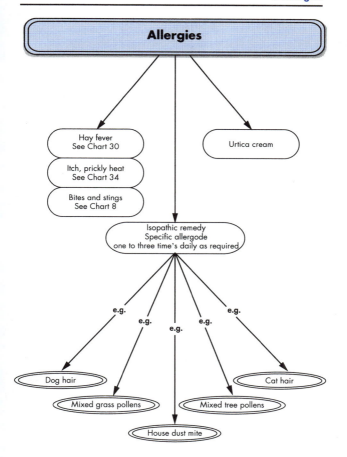

4 Anxiety and shock

- Concurrent use of Rescue Remedy is often useful where mental symptoms predominate (see Chapter 3).
- Relaxation techniques, dietary changes and regular exercise often useful for anxiety.

Homeopathic medicine	Better	Worse	Other
Aconite	In open air, in the evening and at night	Noise and light	Very restless, fear of the future and crowds
Argent nit	In fresh air	From warmth and at night	Fearful and nervous, impulsive
Arnica	Lying down	Motion and cold	Nervous, does not like to be touched or comforted
Arsen alb	Heat and warm drinks	In wet weather and with food	Great fear and despair, restless
Gelsemium	Open air	Excitement and bad news	Stage fright, desire to be quiet and left alone
Ignatia	Movement	In morning and after food	Sad and tearful
Lycopodium	With activity	Heat	Melancholy. Loss of self-confidence. Skin problems
Phosphorus	After sleep and after washing with cold water	After physical or mental exertion	Easily upset. Over-sensitive

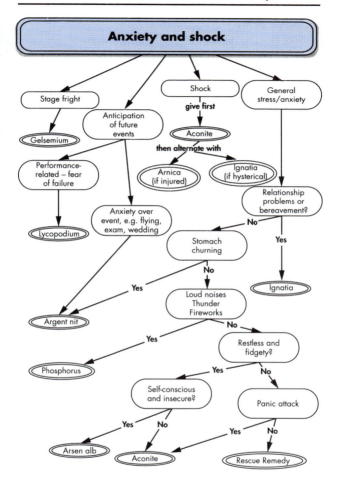

5 Backache

- Arnica 5% gel and Rhus tox/Ruta 5% gel useful topically.
- Non-steroidal anti-inflammatory drugs (oral/topical) and topical rubefacients may be used concurrently but not within 30 minutes of homeopathic medicines.

Homeopathic medicine	Better	Worse	Other
Actaea rac (aka Cimicifuga)	Warm covering	Morning and cold	Very sensitive upper spinal region. Stiffness in neck and back
Ant tart	Sitting up	Lying down and at night	Violent pain in sacro-lumbar region
Arnica	Lying down	Motion	Pain in limbs, difficulty sleeping
Bryonia	Application of cold	Warmth, any motion	Stiffness in small of back and neck region
Hypericum	Rubbing	Cold	Pain radiating up spine and down limbs
Kali carb	Warm weather and gentle movement	Cold weather	General stiffness in back especially in kidney region
Nux vom	Evening	Morning	Pain in lumbar region. Difficulty turning in bed
Rhus tox	Motion and lying on firm surface	Cold weather and at night	Pain between shoulders
Ruta grav	Pressure and lying on back	Lying down and cold	Lumbago, worse before rising

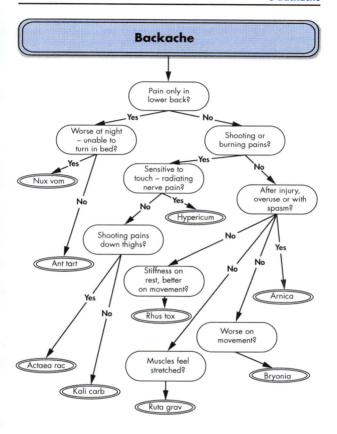

Backache

Pain only in lower back?

— Yes → Worse at night – unable to turn in bed?

— No → Shooting or burning pains?

Worse at night – unable to turn in bed?
- Yes → Nux vom
- No → Ant tart

Shooting or burning pains?
- Yes → Sensitive to touch – radiating nerve pain?
- No → After injury, overuse or with spasm?

Sensitive to touch – radiating nerve pain?
- Yes → Hypericum
- No → Shooting pains down thighs?

Shooting pains down thighs?
- Yes → Actaea rac
- No → Kali carb

After injury, overuse or with spasm?
- Yes → Arnica
- No → Stiffness on rest, better on movement?
- No → Worse on movement?

Stiffness on rest, better on movement?
- Rhus tox
- Muscles feel stretched? → Ruta grav

Worse on movement?
- Bryonia

6 Bedwetting

- Reduce fluid intake in evening.
- Consider cause (e.g. nightmares, stress) and prescribe second medicine if necessary.

Homeopathic medicine	Better	Worse	Other
Argent nit	Fresh air	Warmth and at night	Bad dreams. Pain on urination
Arsen alb	Warmth	Cold	Disturbed and restless sleep
Belladonna	Cool	Hot weather. Mentally active child	Frequent and profuse urination. May shout in sleep
Causticum	Warmth of bed	Cold	Burning sensation in urethra
Equisetum	Reassurance and support to patient	Cold	Pain and tenderness in bladder region
Lycopodium	Uncovered in bed	Heat	Pain in back before urination
Plantago	In the dark	Tobacco smoke	Profuse flow of urine often with pain. Insomnia. Sharp pain in eyes
Pulsatilla	In cool fresh room, uncovered in bed	In warm room. Lying down	Associated with coughing and passing wind

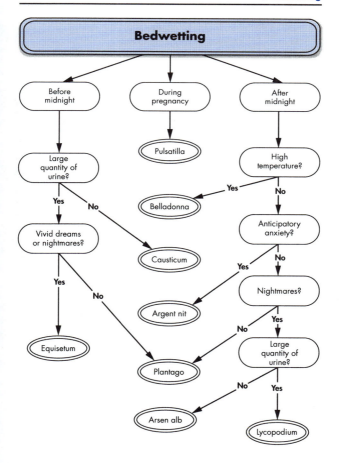

7 Bereavement

- **FIM** – Ignatia for immediate effects of bereavement.
- Rescue Remedy may also be useful.

Homeopathic medicine	Better	Worse	Other
Acid phos	Warmth	From conversation	Headache and confusion Diarrhoea. Cannot collect thoughts
Arsen alb	Heat	In wet weather and cold	Great fear of being left alone
Lachesis	Warmth – wrapped up	After sleep	Restless and talks a lot
Nat mur	In open air	Noise; being consoled	Depression, fright and anger
Pulsatilla	In open air	Heat	Fear of being alone. Weepy
Sepia	After exercise	In cold air	Irritable and anxious, especially in the evening

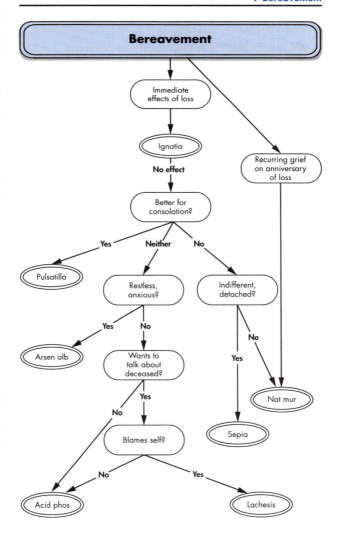

8 Bites and stings

- **FIM** – Apis for bee, wasp and jellyfish stings.
- Apply tinctures neat or diluted tds.
- Apply creams tds.
- If experiencing difficulty breathing, wheezing or heart palpitations, see a doctor immediately.

Homeopathic medicine	Better	Worse	Other
Apis	Application of cold	Heat and pressure	Sore and sensitive, swelling after bite
Cantharis	With rubbing	Touch	Burning pain
Hypericum	With rubbing	In cold. Application of pressure	Also used for crush injuries
Ledum	Cold	At night and from heat	Puncture wounds
Urtica	With rubbing	Touch	Itchy blotches

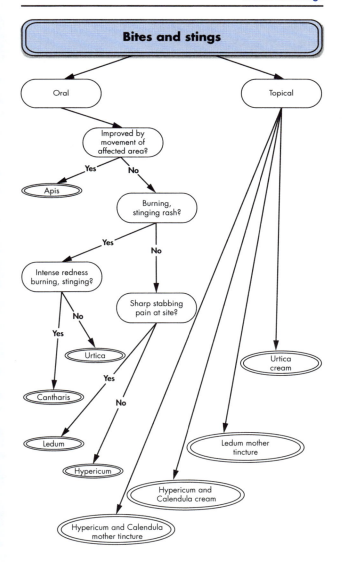

Bites and stings

Oral → Topical

Oral → Improved by movement of affected area?

- Yes → Apis
- No → Burning, stinging rash?
  - Yes → Intense redness burning, stinging?
    - Yes → Cantharis
    - No → Urtica
  - No → Sharp stabbing pain at site?
    - Yes → Ledum
    - No → Hypericum

Intense redness burning, stinging? → Ledum

Topical → Urtica cream

Topical → Ledum mother tincture

Topical → Hypericum and Calendula cream

Topical → Hypericum and Calendula mother tincture

9 Problems associated with breastfeeding

- Application of Hypericum/Calendula 5% cream to nipples between feeds may be beneficial.
- Breastfeeding or expressing should be continued despite acute symptoms as this will help to empty the breast and may contribute to alleviation of symptoms.

Homeopathic medicine	Better	Worse	Other
Acid nit	Steady pressure on breast	Evening and night and in hot weather	Headache; halitosis
Belladonna	Pressure, cool air and rest	Exertion and motion	Vagina dry and hot
Borax	Holding painful part with hand	Downward pressure on breast; warm weather	During nursing, pain in the opposite breast
Bryonia	With pressure on breast and rest	Warmth, motion and touch	Breasts hot, painful and hard
Chamomilla	In mild weather and for application of cold	With heat	Sensitive, irritable, often thirsty; inflamed nipples
Lac caninum	Cold	In the morning and for touch	Prone to mastitis and backache
Lac defloratum	With warm covering	Cold	Prone to constipation
Phytolacca	Warmth	Exposure to damp, cold weather	Severe stinging in breasts
Silica	Warmth	Cold	Nipples very sore
Staphisagria	Lying on back	Cold and motion	Irritability

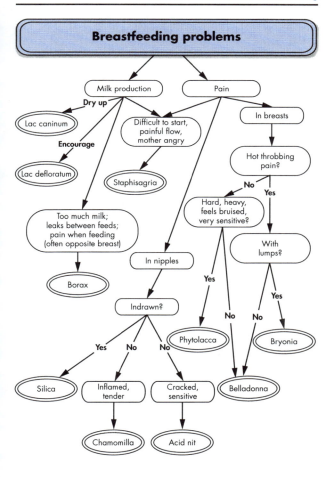

10 Bruising

- **FIM** – Arnica.
- Arnica may be taken tds starting 24–48 h before a surgical or dental procedure.
- Arnica 5% cream or gel is very effective, but do not use on broken skin.
- Ruta 5% ointment, Hypericum 5% ointment and Rhus/Ruta 5% gel may also be effective.

Homeopathic medicine	Better	Worse	Other
Arnica	Lying down	With heat and touch	Black and blue with pain. Patient does not like comforting
Bellis perennis	With local application of cold	With heat and on left side	May be associated with boils
Hamamelis	Rest	In warm, moist air	Also used for varicose veins
Hypericum	With rubbing	In cold	Often involves blood and pain in digits
Ledum	Cold	Warmth	Bruising lasts for some time
Ruta grav	Warmth and scratching	Over-exertion and cold	May be associated with soft tissue injury
Symphytum	Warmth	Touch	May be associated with bone injury

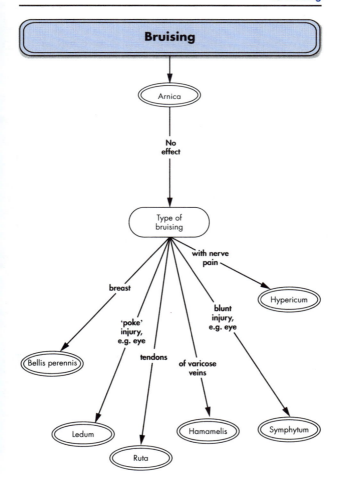

11 Burns

- Hypericum/Calendula tincture useful topically – dilute 5 drops into 100 ml boiled and cooled water and clean the area. This solution may also be used to impregnate a dressing.
- 'Burn' ointment (a product containing mixture of ingredients and available from several manufacturers) may also be used topically in most cases, particularly on the painful outside edges of the burn.
- Sol is a remedy that is not found in all materia medicas. It is made by exposing alcohol to sunlight and when taken orally is useful for sunburn.

Homeopathic medicine	Better	Worse	Other
Aconite	In open air	In warm atmosphere	Red, hot, swollen and burning with numbness
Belladonna	Application of light covering	Touch and heat	Dry, hot and swollen skin with rash
Cantharis	Application of cold	Touch	Scalds and burns
Causticum	Cold drinks	Change of atmosphere	Very painful burns
Sol	Out of sun and cool atmosphere	In warm atmosphere and touch	Sunburn. Can be used prior to exposure
Urtica	Lying down quietly	Touch	Erythema with burning and stinging

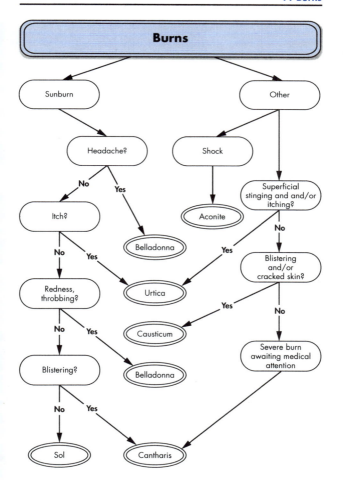

12 Catarrh and sinus problems

- 'Stuffiness' in a baby may respond well to Pulsatilla alone or in conjunction with normal saline nasal drops.
- Inhalations may be used concurrently but should be avoided within 30 minutes of taking the homeopathic remedy.
- If no single medicine is strongly indicated a combination of Kali bich and Pulsatilla 30c given tds for 5–7 days can often be effective.
- Persistent symptoms, especially at night, could be an indication of an allergy, e.g. house dust mite.

Homeopathic medicine	Better	Worse	Other
Arsen iod	Open air	Exertion	Dry and hacking cough
Cinnabaris	Open air	After walking	Hoarseness
Hepar sulph	Moist heat	Cold, dry air	Wheezing, possible association with asthma
Hydrastis	Dry weather	Cold air	Dry, harsh cough
Lachesis	Open air	After sleep	Dry, tickly cough
Kali bich	Heat	Cold	Wheezing on waking. Whooping-type cough
Kali iod	Cold air	Heat	May cause difficulties during the night due to inability to lie down in comfort
Mezereum	Open air	At night	Tightness in chest, may be associated with snoring
Nat mur	Open air	With exertion	Shortness of breath and tickling cough
Pulsatilla	In open air	Heat	Dry cough in evening and at night
Pyrogenium	Heat (hot baths, hot drinks)	Cold and motion	Wheezing
Sticta	In open air	Sudden changes of temperature	Sore throat and dry hacking cough during the night

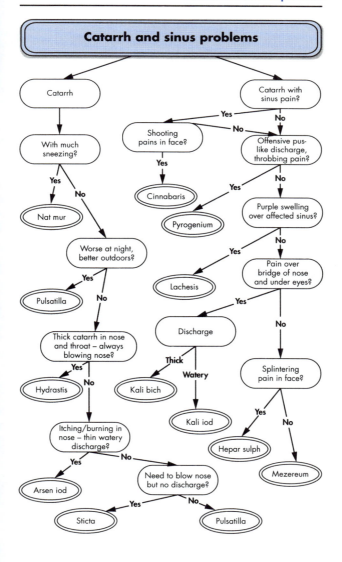

Catarrh and sinus problems

Catarrh

Catarrh with sinus pain?

With much sneezing?

Yes → Nat mur

No → Worse at night, better outdoors?

Yes → Pulsatilla

No → Thick catarrh in nose and throat – always blowing nose?

Yes → Hydrastis

No → Itching/burning in nose – thin watery discharge?

Yes → Arsen iod

No → Need to blow nose but no discharge?

Yes → Sticta

No → Pulsatilla

Catarrh with sinus pain?

Yes → Shooting pains in face?

Yes → Cinnabaris

No → Offensive pus-like discharge, throbbing pain?

Shooting pains in face? → **Yes** → Pyrogenium

Offensive pus-like discharge, throbbing pain?

Yes → Pyrogenium

No → Purple swelling over affected sinus?

Yes → Lachesis

No → Pain over bridge of nose and under eyes?

Yes → Discharge

Discharge → **Thick** → Kali bich

Discharge → **Watery** → Kali iod

No → Splintering pain in face?

Yes → Hepar sulph

No → Mezereum

13 Chickenpox and shingles

- Hypericum/Calendula tincture useful topically for chickenpox – dilute 5 drops into 100 ml boiled and cooled water and apply to spots.
- Calamine lotion may be used concurrently when tincture has absorbed.

Homeopathic medicine	Better	Worse	Other
Ant crud	Open air	In evening	Itching when warm in bed
Ant tart	For sitting up	Lying down and in the warm	Pustular eruptions leaving bluish-red mark
Apis	Keeping cool	Heat	Sore and sensitive, urticaria-like eruptions
Arsen alb	Heat	Cold and scratching	Dry, rough papules
Causticum	Warm weather; gentle motion	Damp, wet weather	Profuse sweat on slight exertion
Hypericum	Lying quietly	Touch	May be associated with diarrhoea
Kalmia	Lying down	Motion	Red, inflamed and painful areas of skin
Mezereum	Open air	At night	May be associated with oozing eruptions
Ranunc bulb	Warm weather	Change of temperature	Burning and intense itching
Rhus tox	Heat	Cold air	Intense itching of skin
Spigelia	Dry air	Touch (pressure of clothes)	Restless sleep with frequent awakening

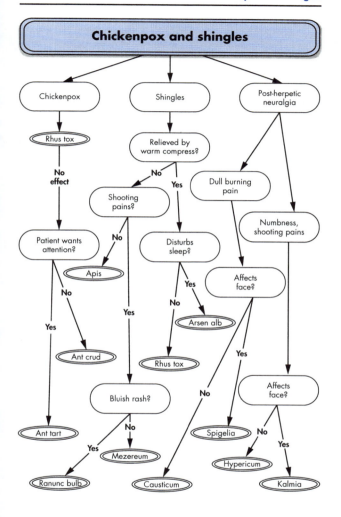

14 Cold and flu

- For prevention – Influenzinum/Bacillinum combination sarcode once daily on same day each week, increasing to od every day if at risk and tds if experiencing acute symptoms.
- If appropriate, herbal Echinacea can be very valuable to boost the immune system – 825 mg daily (adult dose).
- Inhalations and rubs may be used concurrently but should be avoided within 30 minutes of homeopathic treatment.

Homeopathic medicine	Better	Worse	Other
Aconite	In open air	In warm room and at night	Red inflamed eyes, coryza. Swollen tongue. Sore throat. Hoarse, croupy cough
Allium cepa	In open air and cold room	In evening in warm room	Acrid nasal discharge and bland eye secretions. Eyes red. Headache
Arsen iod	Open air and after food	In dry weather and exertion	Slight hacking cough. Thin watery discharge from nose
Belladonna	Sitting up	Touch and noise and lying down	Hot and flushed appearance. Nasal coryza. Tickling dry cough
Bryonia	Rest and cold	Warmth and motion	Coryza with headache
Eupatorium perf	Lying on back	In cold air	Coryza with sneezing. Hoarseness and cough
Euphrasia	In cool	In evening and for warmth	Eye symptoms, acid lacrimation, bland coryza. Frequent yawning
Ferrum phos	Lying down	Night and with cold and motion	Tickling cough, sore chest, sore throat. Prone to nose bleed
Gelsemium	In open air	Damp weather and excitement	Difficulty in swallowing, halitosis
Merc sol	Moderate temperature and rest	Worse at night and warm room and warm bed	Bluish, red, sore throat. Thick discharge from eyes. Back pain
Nat mur	In open air	In warm room and lying down	Fluent coryza, 1–3 days then stopped-up nose, burning in eyes
Nux vom	After sleep	In the morning	Nose stuffed up especially at night. Eyes sensitive to light
Rhus tox	Change of position and stretching of limbs	During sleep at night	Sore throat, sneezing and coryza especially after getting wet. Dry cough

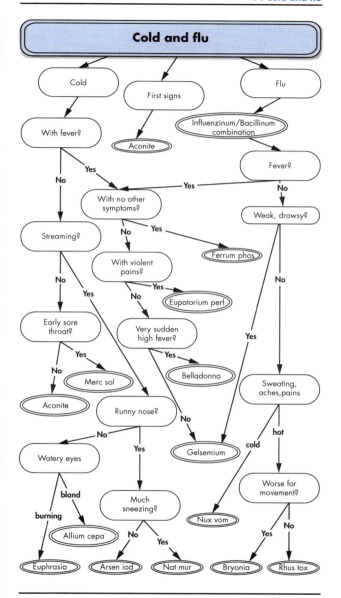

15 Cold sores

- For prevention – Herpes simplex nosode 30c once or twice daily, increasing to tds if required for treatment.
- Hypericum/Calendula 5% cream/ointment useful topically.
- Hypericum and Calendula tincture has been used topically but may sting on application because of the alcohol content.

Homeopathic medicine	Better	Worse	Other
Arsen alb	Heat and warm drinks	Cold and cold drinks	May be associated with gums that bleed easily and also dry rough skin
Capsicum	Heat	Open air	May be associated with halitosis and burning on tip of tongue
Hepar sulph	Damp weather	Dry, cold air	Gums and mouth may bleed easily. May also suffer from skin abscesses
Nat mur	Open air	Warm room	Lips and corner of mouth dry and cracked; also crack in middle of lower lip
Rhus tox	Warm dry weather	Cold wet weather	Sore gums, red and cracked tongue
Sempervivum	None recorded	None recorded	Sore and painful tongue with ulcers that bleed easily. Herpes

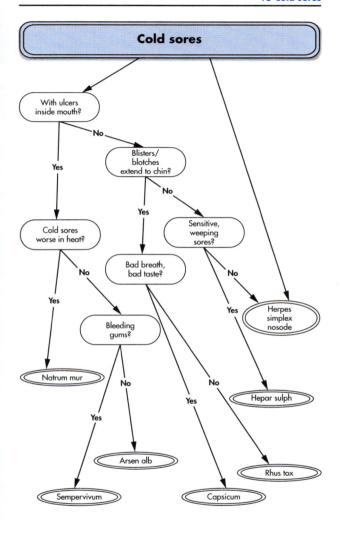

Cold sores

- With ulcers inside mouth?
  - Yes → Cold sores worse in heat?
    - Yes → Natrum mur
    - No → Bleeding gums?
  - No → Blisters/ blotches extend to chin?
    - Yes → Bad breath, bad taste?
    - No → Sensitive, weeping sores?
      - No → Herpes simplex nosode
      - Yes → Hepar sulph

Bleeding gums?
- Yes → Sempervivum
- No → Arsen alb

Bad breath, bad taste?
- Yes → Capsicum
- No → Rhus tox

16 Colic

- **FIM** – for babies, usually Colocynth (or consider Chamomilla if teething).
- The medicine should be given directly to the baby, not the mother, as it is not known to be expressed in breast milk.
- Persistent colic that fails to respond to treatment in a bottlefed baby might be eased by a change of feeding formula. In a breastfed baby, a change in the mother's diet may help.
- Lactase enzyme may be given in the milk concurrently

Homeopathic medicine	Better	Worse	Other
Belladonna	Standing up	Lying down	Associated with loss of appetite, nausea, vomiting and abdominal distension
Carbo veg	After belching	Lying down and in the evening	Abdominal pain and stomach cramps
Chamomilla	Fasting	Night	Distended abdomen, flatulence
Colocynth	Warmth	Anger	Abdominal pain causing patient to bend double
Dioscorea	Standing up in open air	Night and lying down	Abdominal pain that changes location and belching
Nux vom	After sleep	After eating	Sour taste and nausea in morning. Flatulence, distension, spasmodic colic

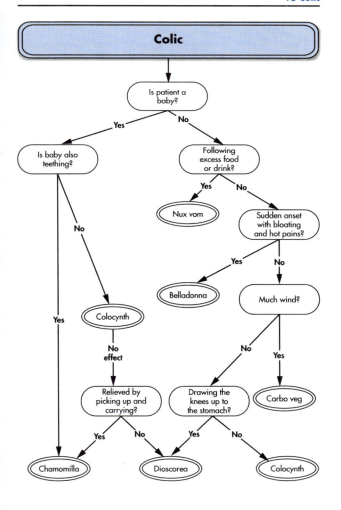

17 Constipation

- If there is no clear medicine indicated, Sulphur 30c in the morning and Nux vom 30c at night for 3 days may be effective.
- Conventional medicine and suppositories may be used concurrently.
- Patient should increase intake of fluids and dietary fibre.

Homeopathic medicine	Better	Worse	Other
Alumina	In open air and after cool wash	In morning and warm room	Colic
Hydrastis	Warm covering	At night	Sore feeling in stomach, white swollen tongue
Nux vom	After sleep	In morning	Very irritable, nausea in morning and after eating. Flatulence
Plumbum met	After physical exertion	At night	Excessive colic
Silica	Warmth	In morning	Abdominal pain and colic
Sulphur	In open air and after activity	At night and in bed	Abdomen sensitive to pressure. Itching and burning of anus. Loss of appetite

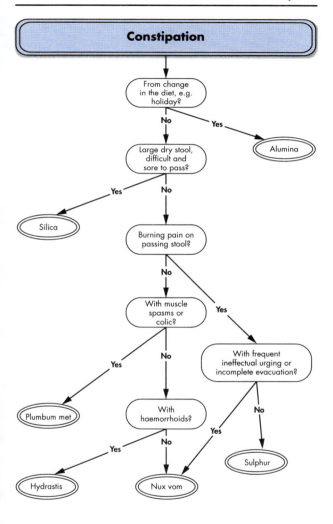

18 Cough

- For persistent coughs that seem unresponsive, a course of Tuberculinum bovinum 200 (Tub bov) night/morning/night may also be beneficial.
- A persistent cough, especially at night, could be an indication of chronic disease or an allergy, e. g. house dust mite (see Chart 3, Allergies).

Homeopathic medicine	Better	Worse	Other
Aconite	In open air	In warm room and from dry, cold winds	Hoarse, dry, croupy cough
Ant tart	Sitting up	In evening and lying down	Hoarse cough with burning sensation in chest
Belladonna	Sitting up	In a draught and lying down	Tickling, short, dry cough
Bryonia	In cool	With activity, after eating and drinking	Dry, hacking cough
Drosera	When active	At night	Spasmodic, dry, irritating cough
Hepar sulph	Warmth	Draught and activity	Hoarseness, with loss of voice
Ipecac	Rest	Warmth	Frequent coughing. Croup. Often associated with coryza and sneezing
Phosphorus	Physical exertion, talking, evening	Lying on right side, fresh air	Hoarseness with dry tickling in the throat. Cough made worse by talking
Pulsatilla	Open air, cold food and drinks	Heat	Urine may be emitted with cough. Expectoration thick and greenish
Spongia	Warmth	In dry, cold wind	Dry, barking, croupy cough. May be associated with bronchial catarrh
Stannum met	Lying down	When using voice	Hoarse cough, sorer chest, may be associated with colic

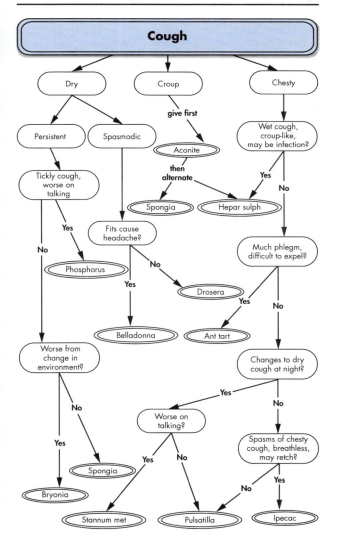

19 Cramp

- **FIM**: at night for restless legs, Zincum met; for leg cramp, Cuprum met. The indicated medicine should be taken in the 30c potency 1 hour before bed, at bedtime and again if wakened.
- The importance of increasing fluids and reducing caffeine intake, especially in the evening, should be stressed.

Homeopathic medicine	Better	Worse	Other
Argent nit	Fresh air and cold	Warmth and at night	May be associated with nausea and passing wind. Also colic
Arnica	Lying down	Heat	Wind and pain in stomach
Bryonia	Cold	Warmth	Nausea and thirst, abdominal pain, constipation
Chamomilla	Heat	At night	Belching and biliousness. Abdominal distension
Cuprum met	Cold drinks	Cold air	Intermittent colic
Gelsemium	Continued motion	After emotion or excitement	Cramp in muscles of forearm. Difficulty sleeping
Mag phos	Warmth and bending double	Cold and night	Windy colic. Weakness in arms and hands
Rhus tox	In warmth and during motion	At night and during rest	Pain in joints and between shoulders
Verat alb	Walking and warmth	Night	Soreness and tenderness of joints. Sciatica
Zinc met	Rubbing	Open air and after food	Twitching of muscles. Chilblains

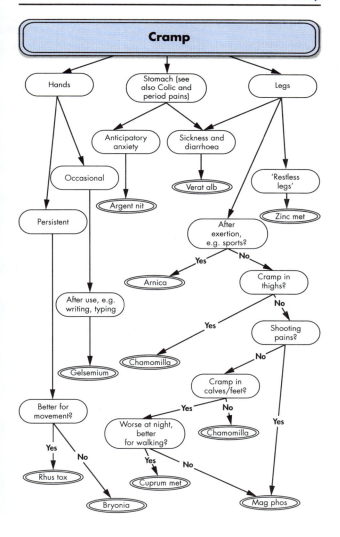

20 Diarrhoea

- **FIM** – Arsen alb.
- Electrolyte replacement therapy may be used concurrently.
- Symptoms may have origins in anxiety, excitement or fear (see Chart 4, Anxiety and shock).

Homeopathic medicine	Better	Worse	Other
Acid phos	Keeping warm	After exertion	Distended abdomen. White, watery diarrhoea; much wind
Aloe soc	Cool atmosphere	Early morning and in hot dry weather	Sense of insecurity when passing wind. Lumpy, watery stool
Argent nit	After belching and in fresh air	Night and warmth. Cold food	Colic. Watery, green stools. Abdominal distension. Anxiety
Arsen alb	Warm drinks	After cold drinks and food and at night	Nausea and vomiting
Chamomilla	After fasting	Heat and at night	Distended abdomen. Hot, green, watery stool with colic
Colocynth	Warmth	Emotional upset	Abdominal pain, colic and cramps
Ipecac	After passage of stool	After eating and at night	Dark-green stools with mucus
Podophyllum	Evening and when bending forward	Early morning and hot weather	Abdominal distension, rumbling and shifting of flatus. Nausea
Sulphur	Dry, warm weather	At rest. Standing	Drinks a lot, eats little. Itching and burning of anus
Verat alb	Warmth	At night	Abdominal pain and cramps in legs

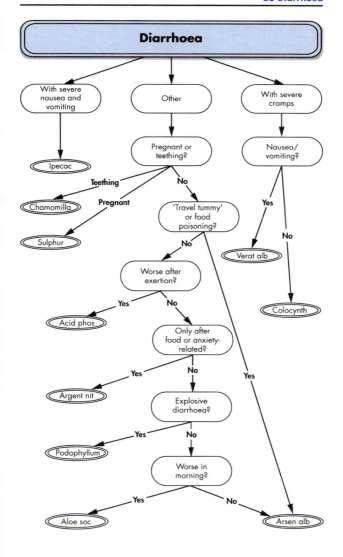

21 Ear problems

- For recurring ear problems, a constitutional medicine may be more suitable – a detailed consultation would be required. Consider referral.
- Conventional ear drops may be used concurrently.
- Verbascum mother tincture applied topically may be appropriate.

Homeopathic medicine	Better	Worse	Other
Aconite	In open air	In warm room and lying on affected side	External ear often hot, red and swollen. Very sensitive to noise
Acid sal	None recorded	Night and in cold air	Deafness with vertigo
Apis	In open air	Heat	External ear red and inflamed
Belladonna	After rest	Touch and noise	Pain in middle and external ear. Sensitive to loud noises
Carbo sulph	In open air	In warm, damp weather	Headache and dizziness. Impaired hearing
Chamomilla	In damp weather	Heat, emotional upset and touch	Earache with soreness
China	In open air and lying down	In cold and draughts	Impaired hearing, sensitive to noise
Graphites	Dark	Warmth	Headache in the morning on wakening
Hepar sulph	In damp weather	Slightest draught and cold winds	Whizzing and throbbing in ears
Kali mur	Cold drinks	In open air	May be associated with chronic catarrh
Lycopodium	At night	Heat	May be associated with eczema behind ears. Yellow discharge possible
Pulsatilla	Open air	Heat	External ear swollen and red, bland discharge possible
Pyrogenium	Heat	Cold	Possible loud, ringing noise in ears

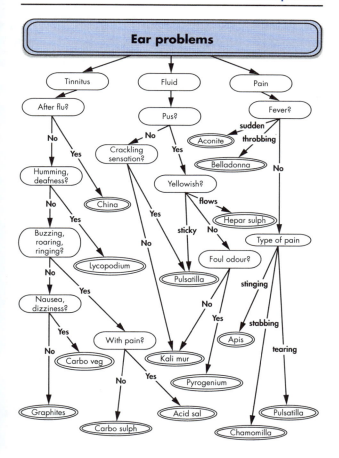

22 Eczema and dermatitis

- Graphites, Rhus tox or Sulphur 5% creams as appropriate may be useful topically.
- For conditions affecting the scalp, Calendula shampoo may be useful.
- Tautodes should be considered where a skin condition has been caused by chemical irritation (see Isopathic medicines in Chapter 3).

Homeopathic medicine	Better	Worse	Other
Arsen alb	Application of heat	In the cold	Itching, burning, dry and rough eruptions
Graphites	In the open air	In the cold	Rough, hard and dry skin
Mezereum	In the open air	At night and with touch	Eczema with itching
Petroleum	In dry weather	In winter	Itching at night, skin dry, rough and cracked
Psorinum	In heat	In changeable weather	Sore pain behind ears, possible discharge from eczema around ears
Rhus tox	In warm	In cold	Pain in ears. Swollen lobules
Sulphur	Dry, warm weather	After washing and with warmth in bed	Burning and itching, worse from scratching. May be associated with pruritis

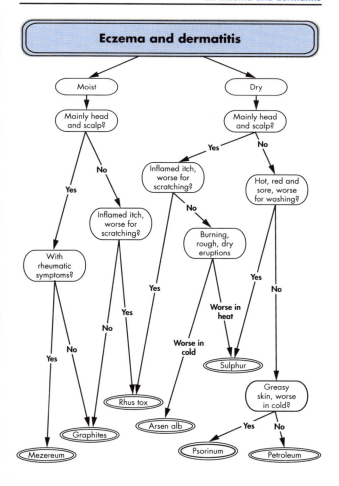

23 Eye problems

- Euphrasia (commonly called 'Eyebright') tincture useful topically – dilute 5 drops into 100 ml boiled and cooled water and bathe. Note: this is not sterile and must not be used undiluted.
- Euphrasia eye drops (sterile) are available at the time of writing as a prescription-only medicine.
- Other unlicensed eye drops are also available.

Homeopathic medicine	Better	Worse	Other
Argent nit	Cold	Night	Blurred vision, eyes photosensitive. Headache
Arnica	Lying down	Touch	Dizzy feeling on closing eyes
Euphrasia	In the dark	In evening and in bright light	Burning and swelling of lids with frequent blinking. Bursting headache
Graphites	In the dark	Warmth and at night	Eyelids red and swollen
Ledum	In cold	Warmth and at night	Burning on margin of lids. Feeling of sand in eyes
Merc sol	In moderate temperature	At night	Burning, acrid discharge. Patients report 'floating black spots'. Vertigo
Pulsatilla	In open air	Heat	Bland discharge, styes, profuse lacrimation
Sabadilla	In warm	In cold	Eyelids red and burning. Eyes water when looking at light, sneezing
Staphisagria	Warmth	After emotional upset	Recurrent styes, corner of eyelids itch
Symphytum	During the day	Pain worse at night	Continual inflammation, profuse lacrimation, pain

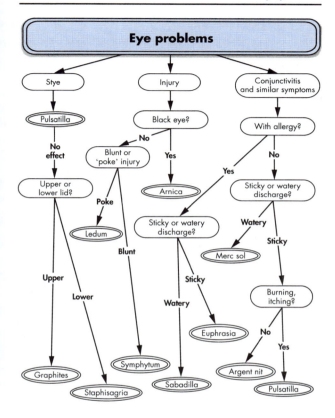

Eye problems

- Stye
  - Pulsatilla
    - **No effect**
    - Upper or lower lid?
      - **Upper** → Graphites
      - **Lower** → Staphisagria

- Injury
  - Black eye?
    - **No** → Blunt or 'poke' injury
      - **Poke** → Ledum
      - **Blunt** → Symphytum
    - **Yes** → Arnica
  - Sticky or watery discharge?
    - **Sticky** → Euphrasia
    - **Watery** → Sabadilla

- Conjunctivitis and similar symptoms
  - With allergy?
    - **Yes** → Sticky or watery discharge?
      - **Watery** → Merc sol
      - **Sticky** → Burning, itching?
        - **No** → Argent nit
        - **Yes** → Pulsatilla
    - **No**

24 Fatigue (acute)

- For prevention of jetlag – Arnica tds on day of departure and arrival and every 2 hours during flight (if awake).
- Homeopathy can also be valuable in *chronic* fatigue – a referral for a detailed consultation would be required.

Homeopathic medicine	Better	Worse	Other
Acid phos	Keeping warm	Exertion	Headache, worse with noise. Eyelids inflamed
Acid pic	Cold air and cold water	With least exertion	Back pain, 'pins and needles' sensation in hands and feet
Arnica	Lying down	Touch	Confusion, wants to be left alone
China	None recorded	When eating and after mental exertion	Sensitive to noise and bitter taste in mouth
Cocculus	Lying on side	During eating and in open air	Suffers from motion sickness
Kali phos	Warmth and rest	Excitement and physical exertion	Headache and vertigo
Merc sol	Moderate temperature	At night	Sweating on head
Scutellaria	Sleep	Over-exertion	Dull headache and nausea
Zinc met	Warm open air and eating	Noise	Violent headache after drinking wine, eyes sore and lacrimating

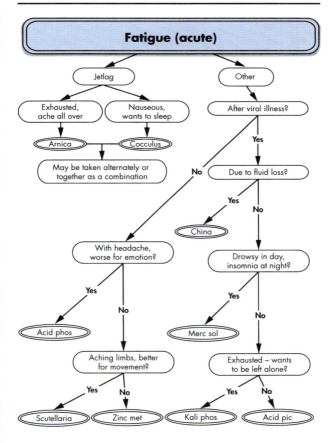

25 Fever

- **FIM** – Belladonna may be the medicine of choice, particularly if the patient is very hot and flushed and the condition came on suddenly.
- Paracetamol and/or ibuprofen may be used concurrently but not within 30 minutes of the homeopathic medicine.

Homeopathic medicine	Better	Worse	Other
Aconite	In open air	In warm room and tobacco smoke	Red, hot and flushed face. Red, dry throat. Nightmares. Cold sweat
Arsen alb	Heat and warm drinks	Cold	Swollen, burning sore throat. High temperature and exhaustion
Baptisia	Drinking liquids and in open air	Heat	Difficulty in swallowing, sore throat, heat all over body
Belladonna	Sitting up	Touch and lying down	High fever, sudden onset. Perspiration on head
Bryonia	Cold	Warmth and motion	Profuse perspiration. May be associated with rheumatic pain
Ferrum phos	Application of cold	Night	May be associated with catarrh
Gelsemium	Open air, drinks	Excitement, bad news	Chilliness up and down back, muscular soreness, perspiration and headache
Merc sol	Moderate temperature and after rest	At night, in warm room and in warm bed	Gastric symptoms. Debility. Profuse perspiration

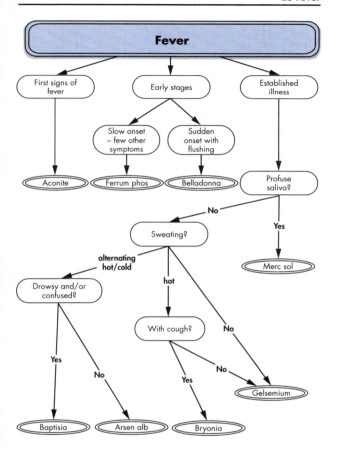

26 Flatulence

- **FIM** – Carbo veg.

Homeopathic medicine	Better	Worse	Other
Argent nit	In fresh air	Warmth and at night	Belching, nausea and retching. Much abdominal distension. Colic
Belladonna	When sitting up	When lying down	Abdominal distension and loss of appetite
Carbo veg	After belching	At night and in open air. After eating fatty food	Stomach feels bloated, belching, abdominal pain
Lycopodium	Motion	In heat or warm room	Bloated feeling after eating small quantities of food. Hiccough
Raphanus	Walking in open air	At night and on waking	Retching and vomiting, loss of appetite

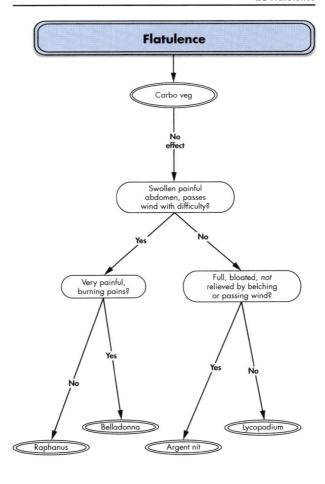

27 Glandular fever

- **FIM** – Glandular fever nosode.
- If appropriate, herbal Echinacea can be very valuable to boost the immune system – 825 mg daily (adult dose).

Homeopathic medicine	Better	Worse	Other
Ailanthus	Hot drinks	Motion	Inflamed and red throat. Hoarse, croupy voice. Often associated with skin conditions
Belladonna	Sitting up	Touch, noise and lying down	High fever, sudden onset
Cistus can	After food	Extremely sensitive to exposure to cold air	Itching in skin, glands inflamed
Merc sol	Moderate temperature and rest	At night and from warm room and warm bed	Profuse perspiration. Salivation

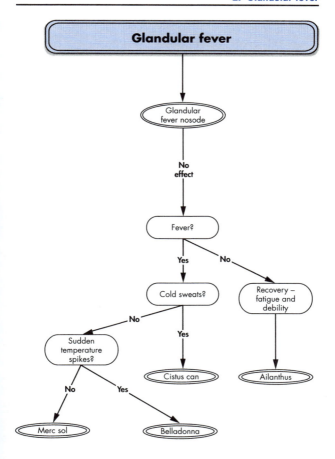

28 Gout

- Importance of diet should be stressed.
- Conventional medication should be continued.

Homeopathic medicine	Better	Worse	Other
Arnica	Lying down	Touch and exertion	Pain in back and limbs. Patient wants to be left alone
Belladonna	When sitting up	When lying down	Shooting pains along limbs, joints swollen, cold extremities
Colchicum	When stooping	In evening and warm weather	Pins and needles in hands and wrists, numb fingertips. Gout in heel
Ledum	Cold	At night	Pains through foot and legs and in joints. Throbbing in right shoulder
Pulsatilla	In open air and from motion	Heat	Pain in limbs that shifts rapidly, knees swollen
Rhus tox	Motion	At night and during rest	Hot, painful, swollen joints
Urtica	None recorded	Cold, moist air and from touch	Pain in ankles and wrists

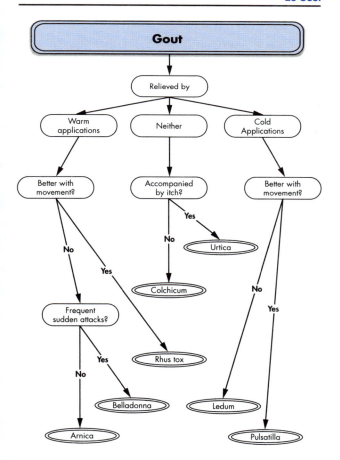

29 Haemorrhoids

- Hamamelis 5% cream useful topically.
- Conventional medicine and suppositories may be used concurrently.
- Usual referral criteria apply.

Homeopathic medicine	Better	Worse	Other
Acid nit	None recorded	In the evening and at night	Great straining but little passage of stools. Constipation
Aesculus	Cool, open air	In morning	Much pain after stool. Painful haemorrhoids; large, hard, dry stools
Aloe soc	Cold	In early morning and summer heat	Lumpy, watery stool with soreness in rectum after passing
Baryta carb	None recorded	In cold weather	Constipation with hard stools
Causticum	After gentle activity	In evening and after passing stool	Soft and small stool, expelled with much difficulty
Collinsonia	Heat	Slightest excitement	Aching feeling in anus, dry stools
Hamamelis	Rest and lying down	Warm air and at night	Sore haemorrhoids, may bleed profusely
Nux vom	In the evening	In the morning	Constipated with ineffectual urging

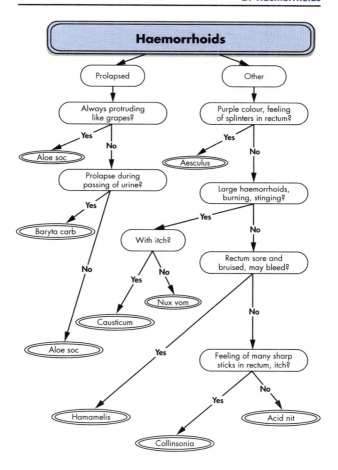

30 Hay fever

- **FIM** – Mixed grass pollen (MGP) 30c up to tds as required.
- Try MGP first, moving to other medicines if effect not satisfactory. Medicines may be co-administered or prepared as a bespoke combination medicine depending on presenting symptoms.
- See also Chart 3, Allergies.

Homeopathic medicine	Better	Worse	Other
Allium cepa	In open air and in cold room	In evening, in warm room	Hacking cough, sneezing, copious discharge from nose
Ambrosia	Cold air	Warm room and in presence of other people	Watery coryza, eyes burning
Ammon mur	In open air	In the morning	Acrid nasal discharge. Skin itching in evening
Arundo	Not recorded	In the evening and with motion	May be associated with eczema. Burning and itching of eyes and nostrils
Euphrasia	In the dark	In the evening	Eyes red and sore, acrid lacrimation, bland coryza
Gelsemium	In open air	In damp weather	Sneezing, watery nasal discharge
Sabadilla	When wrapped up and in open air	In the cold	Spasmodic sneezing with runny nose

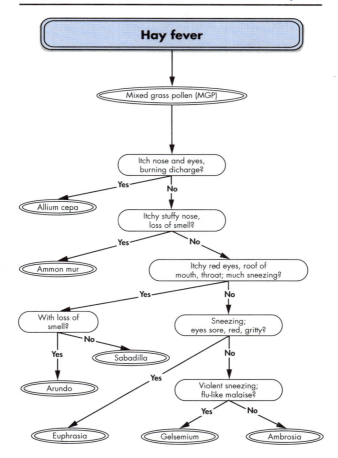

31 Headache and migraine

- Relaxation techniques, dietary changes and regular exercise often useful.
- For frequently recurring symptoms, a constitutional medicine may be more suitable – a detailed consultation would be required.
- The site and intensity of pain are important in identifying the correct medicine.

Homeopathic medicine	Better	Worse	Other
Belladonna	Sitting down	Noise and lying down	Often fever, pain in forehead. Sudden onset
Bryonia	In cold	Motion	Vertigo, nausea and faintness on rising
Glonoine	Open air, elevating head	In the sun or beside open fire. Lying down	Abnormalities of vision
Ignatia	Change of position	Tobacco smoke	Congestive headaches following anger or grief
Iris vers	Continued motion	In evening and during night	Frontal headache with nausea. Ringing in the ears. Facial neuralgia
Lachesis	In warm atmosphere	After sleep	May be associated with sun. Vertigo
Lycopodium	Motion and warm food and drink	Headache worse early evening and lying down	Throbbing headache especially after coughing
Nat mur	In open air	Noise and in a warm room	Blinding headache
Nux vom	While at rest and in the evening	Morning and after eating	Frontal and congestive headache. Eyes photosensitive. Stuffed up nose
Sanguinaria	Lying down and sleep	On right side	Pain in the back of the head, flushed face. May be associated with sun
Silica	Warmth	In the morning	Pain over most of head. Aversion to light. Very sensitive to cold air
Spigelia	Lying down	Touch and noise	Throbbing pain in front of head
Staphisagria	During night and warmth	Emotional upset	Associated with eye symptoms
Thuja	Warmth and motion	At night from heat of bed	Left-sided headache may be associated with chronic otitis and catarrh

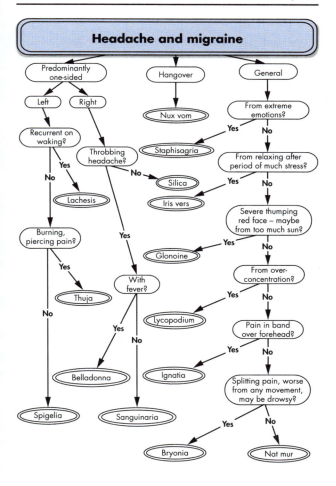

32 Hot flushes

- Often the best long-term dosage regimen is the indicated medicine in the 6c potency given tds for 3 days then bd. This may be increased to 12c on follow-up or supplemented by a further supply of the indicated medicine in 30c for acute symptoms.
- Conventional medication, e. g. HRT (hormone replacement therapy) should be continued unless stopped by the prescribing doctor.
- See also Chart 36, Menopause.

Homeopathic medicine	Better	Worse	Other
Amyl nit	Cool air	Anxiety	Facial flushing with anxiety and palpitation. Hiccough and yawning
Aurum met	Cool, open air	At night	Vaginal discomfort and uterine problems
Belladonna	Sitting up	Lying down	May be associated with painful breasts
Glonoine	Open air. Elevating head	Lying down	Often associated with backache
Graphites	Wrapping up	At night	Constipation. Pale and scanty menses. Weakness in back. Swollen breasts
Jaborandi	Cool atmosphere	At start of menses	Backache and often much coughing. Profuse sweating and nausea
Lachesis	Open air, cold drinks and loosening clothes	Pressure from clothes and after sleep	Palpitation, flushes of heat and fainting. Sciatica. Painful breasts
Pulsatilla	Open air and motion	Heat and towards evening	Chilliness and nausea, pain in the back, diarrhoea
Sepia	Exercise and warmth of bed	Morning and evening	Morning sickness, pain in vagina, back pain
Sulphur	Dry, warm weather	At rest and from warmth in bed	Burning sensation in vagina, cracked nipples

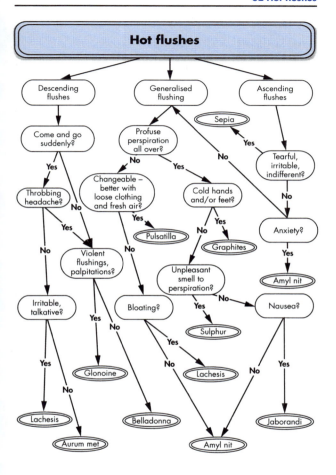

33 Injury

- **FIM** – any injury will usually respond to Arnica.
- Topical treatments include Arnica, Calendula, Hypericum Calendula.
- See also Chart 10, Bruising, Chart 50, Sports injuries and Chart 51, Sprains and strains.
- Arnica and Rhus tox/Ruta gel can be useful topically.
- For fractures: Symphytum 30c should be taken tds for no more than 10 days.

Homeopathic medicine	Better	Worse	Other
Aconite	In open air	In warm room	Anxiety and fear. Vomiting, mouth dry and tingling
Arnica	Lying down	Touch	Bruising. Skin itching and burning
Hypericum	Lying quietly	In cold	Blood and crush injuries, particularly involving digits
Symphytum	By changing position and applying heat	At night	Bone involvement. Numbness in palms of hand and soles of feet

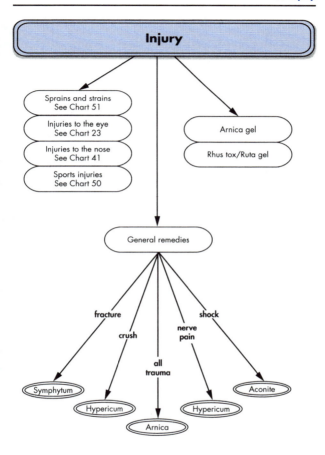

Injury

- Sprains and strains
  See Chart 51
- Injuries to the eye
  See Chart 23
- Injuries to the nose
  See Chart 41
- Sports injuries
  See Chart 50

- Arnica gel
- Rhus tox/Ruta gel

General remedies

fracture — Symphytum

crush — Hypericum

all trauma — Arnica

nerve pain — Hypericum

shock — Aconite

34 Itch

- Urtica 5% cream useful topically – may be kept in fridge for maximum relief.
- For prevention of prickly heat, Sol may be taken in the 30c potency bd starting 1 week before exposure, increasing to tds and used concurrently with Urtica 5% cream if acute symptoms are experienced.
- See also Chart 3, Allergies.
- Sol is a remedy that is not found in all materia medicas. It is made by exposing alcohol to sunlight. When taken orally it is useful for itching and burning skin following exposure to sun. See Chart 11, Burns.

Homeopathic medicine	Better	Worse	Other
Agaricus	Movement	In cold air	Often associated with chilblains and small pimples. Restless sleep causes itching and burning skin
Apis	In open air	Heat and touch	Stinging pain and oedema in extremities. Hives with itching
Nat mur	In open air	Heat	Dry eruptions on skin. Pain in back. Hives, itching after exertion
Rhus tox	Motion and in warm dry weather	During sleep	Red, swollen, itching skin with vesicles. Restlessness
Sol	In cool	In direct sunlight	Associated with exposure to sun
Urtica	Lying down	Cold air	Urticarial rash. Erythema with burning and stinging. Itching of scrotum

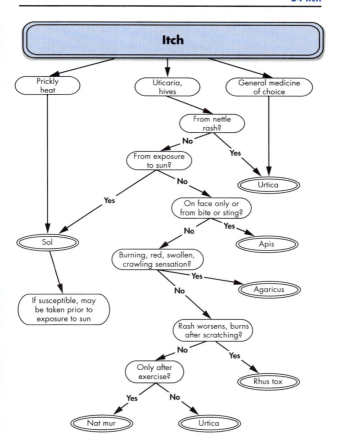

35 Problems associated with labour

- Arnica tds – start 2 days before due date (or as soon as possible) and continue until recovery.
- Caulophyllum should be taken bd starting 10 days before due date to ease passage of labour – stop when labour begins. If being used when progression of labour stops, the medicine should be taken hourly for three doses or until progression resumes.
- Hypericum/Calendula tincture useful – add 10 drops to a bath to relieve soreness from stitches, tearing or episiotomy.

Homeopathic medicine	Better	Worse	Other
Aconite	Lying down	In warm room	Worry and anxiety. Red, inflamed eyes
Arnica	Lying down	Least touch	Used to reduce bruising and pain
Bellis perennis	Gentle movement	In warmth of bed	Trauma of the pelvic organs. Varicose veins in pregnancy, difficulty in walking. Wakes early in morning
Caulophyllum	Warmth	Open air	Spasmodic and severe pains. Dyspepsia
Chamomilla	With cold application	Heat	Where labour pains spasmodic, patient intolerant of pain. May be bloody discharge. Often irritable dry cough
Ipecac	Closing eyes, rest	Warmth	Irritable and anxious. Continuous nausea. Labour pains spasmodic and cutting across from left to right
Kali phos	Warmth and rest	Worry and physical exertion	Labour pains continual but of low intensity
Lac caninum	Cold and with cold drinks	Morning or evening	Erratic labour pains
Lac defloratum	After food	Warmth	Throbbing pains with nausea and vomiting, constipation. Associated with poor nutrition

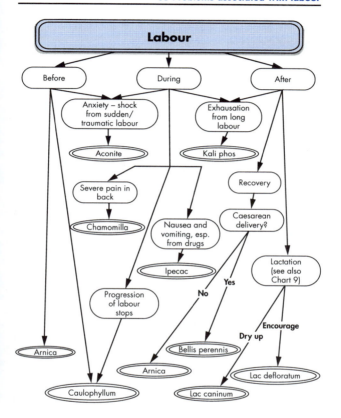

36 Problems associated with the menopause

- Hamamelis 5% cream may also be useful for varicose veins – apply bd.
- Conventional medication, e. g. HRT, should be continued unless stopped by the prescribing doctor.
- See also Chart 32, Hot flushes.

Homeopathic medicine	Better	Worse	Other
Actaea rac (aka Cimicifuga)	Warmth and after food	In the morning and in the cold	Pain in ovarian region, nausea and vomiting. Headache associated with worry
Arnica	Lying down	With touch and motion	Sore nipples
Caulophyllum	Warmth	Open air	Spasmodic and severe pains in abdominal region. Thrush
Hamamelis	In open air and rest	In warm, moist air	Bearing down pain in back, vagina irritable and tender, sore nipples
Ignatia	While eating	In the morning	Disinterest in sexual activity, dry spasmodic cough. Very light sleep
Pulsatilla	Open air and motion	Heat	Patient fears to be alone and likes sympathy. Dyspepsia after a meal. Amenorrhoea

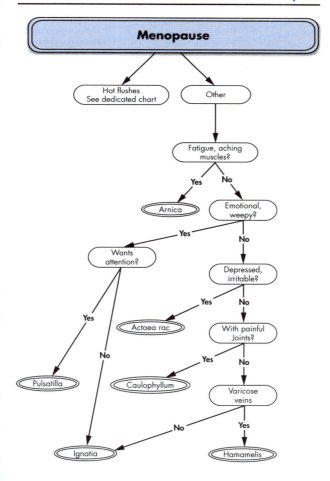

37 Morning sickness in pregnancy

- Symptoms may occur at any time of day and may or may not persist.
- Acupressure wrist bands are also effective in some cases.
- No adverse drug reactions or untoward effects on fetus noted in the homeopathic literature.

Homeopathic medicine	Better	Worse	Other
Aletris	After passing wind	None recorded	Small amounts of food can cause dyspepsia, flatulence and colic. Fainting spells
Amygdalus per	None recorded	None recorded	Constant nausea and vomiting. Occasional blood in urine
Apomorphinum	Not recorded	After eating	Constipation, insomnia, vertigo. Vomiting accompanied by increased secretion of sweat and saliva
Cocculus	Lying quietly	After eating, loss of sleep and motion	Abdominal distension with wind
Cucurbita pep	Not recorded	After eating	Indicated for intense nausea and vomiting of pregnancy
Ipecac	Cool air	Lying down and warmth, also nausea worse from looking at moving objects	Constant nausea and vomiting, much saliva and hiccoughs
Nux vom	When resting	In the morning and after eating	Sour taste in the mouth and stomach pain. Flatulence
Pulsatilla	In open air and with a cold drink	Heat and after eating, especially rich, fatty food	Abdominal distension, heartburn
Sepia	After exercise and sleep	Morning and evening	Nausea at smell and sight of food
Symphoricarpus	Lying on back	During motion	Constipation, gastric disturbances

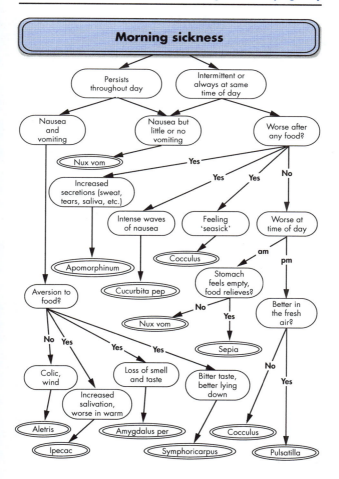

38 Mouth problems

- **FIM** – Merc sol for most acute mouth problems.
- Hypericum/Calendula tincture useful as a mouthwash – dilute 10 drops in 100 ml boiled/cooled water and use up to qds as required.
- Herbal Echinacea can benefit if patient suffers persistent ulcers – 825 mg daily (adult dose) if appropriate.

Homeopathic medicine	Better	Worse	Other
Acid nit	Hot drinks	Evening and night	Bleeding of gums, ulcers on soft palate, burning in throat
Belladonna	Cold drinks	Heat and warm drinks	Throbbing pain in teeth, gumboils, tongue swollen, dry throat with enlarged tonsils
Borax	Cold weather	Warm weather	Mouth hot and tender, ulcers may bleed, gumboils and bitter taste
Bryonia	Warmth	With cold drinks	Lips dry and cracked, excessive thirst, bitter taste in the mouth, dry throat
Hydrastis	In dry air	In cold air	Peppery taste in mouth, tongue white, swollen and large. Gums dark red and swollen
Kreosotum	Warmth	In open air	Halitosis and bitter taste in mouth. Lips red and bleeding
Merc sol	Moderate temperature	In warm atmosphere and in warm bed	Increased saliva, halitosis, burning sensation in throat
Phosphorus	With cold food and after sleep	With warm food and drink	Dry tongue and toothache
Silica	Warmth	Cold	Pain on swallowing and gumboils

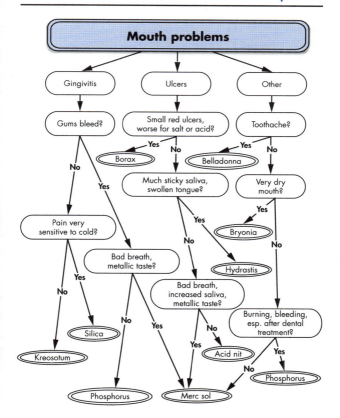

Mouth problems

Gingivitis
- Gums bleed?
  - No → Pain very sensitive to cold?
    - No → Kreosotum
    - Yes → Silica
  - Yes → Bad breath, metallic taste?
    - Yes → Phosphorus
    - No → Merc sol

Ulcers
- Small red ulcers, worse for salt or acid?
  - Yes → Borax
  - No → Much sticky saliva, swollen tongue?
    - Yes → Hydrastis
    - No → Bad breath, increased saliva, metallic taste?
      - Yes → Merc sol
      - No → Acid nit

Other
- Toothache?
  - Yes → Belladonna
  - No → Very dry mouth?
    - Yes → Bryonia
    - No → Burning, bleeding, esp. after dental treatment?
      - Yes → Phosphorus
      - No → Merc sol

39 Nappy rash

- Both topical and oral treatment may be used concurrently.
- Use of barrier cream may be appropriate after topical treatment.

Homeopathic medicine	Better	Worse	Other
Croton tig	Removing nappy	Touch and washing	Intense itching; pustular eruptions. Dark orange-coloured urine
Merc sol	Moderate temperature	At night	Constantly moist skin, cold clammy sweat on legs at night. Greenish, slimy stool
Rhus tox	In warmth	During sleep	Red, swollen, itching skin. Dark-coloured urine. Diarrhoea, with mucus
Sulphur	Lying on right side	Over-warmth in bed	Frequent urination, especially at night. Redness around anus with itching

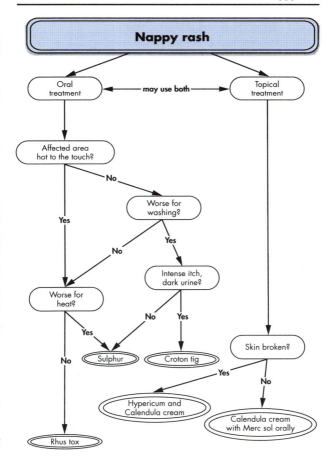

40 Nausea and vomiting

- **FIM** – Nux vom (nausea); Ipecac (vomiting).
- Electrolyte replacement therapy may be used concurrently.

Homeopathic medicine	Better	Worse	Other
Anacardium	Eating	Between meals	Belching, nausea and vomiting, abdominal pain and constipation
Ant crud	During rest	In the evening	Thirst in evening and night, heartburn. Desire for acids and pickles
Arsen alb	Warm drinks	After food	Cannot bear sight or smell of food, great thirst, retching, heartburn
Ipecac	Hot drinks	Lying down	Mouth moist with much saliva, constant nausea and vomiting, hiccoughs
Nux vom	After rest	After eating particularly spicy food	Sour taste and nausea after eating, belching. Ravenous hunger
Pulsatilla	After cold food and drinks	Rich, fatty food and after eating	Belching, taste of food remains a long time, bitter taste, flatulence, heartburn

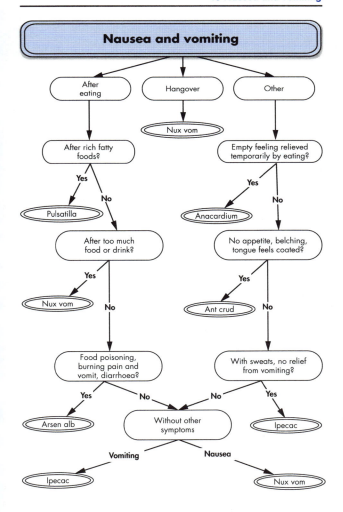

Nausea and vomiting

After eating

Hangover
→ Nux vom

Other

After rich fatty foods?
- **Yes** → Pulsatilla
- **No** → After too much food or drink?
  - **Yes** → Nux vom
  - **No** → Food poisoning, burning pain and vomit, diarrhoea?
    - **Yes** → Arsen alb
    - **No** → Without other symptoms

Empty feeling relieved temporarily by eating?
- **Yes** → Anacardium
- **No** → No appetite, belching, tongue feels coated?
  - **Yes** → Ant crud
  - **No** → With sweats, no relief from vomiting?
    - **No** → Without other symptoms
    - **Yes** → Ipecac

Without other symptoms
- **Vomiting** → Ipecac
- **Nausea** → Nux vom

41 Nosebleed

- If no medicine is clearly indicated, try Phosphorus first.
- For recurring nosebleeds, conventional treatment or a constitutional medicine may be more suitable – a referral would be required.

Homeopathic medicine	Better	Worse	Other
Agaricus	Warm	In open and cold weather	Particularly in older people. Internal and external nasal itching, spasmodic sneezing
Arnica	Lying down	Touch and motion	After coughing fit
Belladonna	Sitting up	Lying down	Red, flushed face, tingling in tip of nose
Ferrum phos	Application of cold	At night	First stage of head cold, bright red blood, face flushed, cheeks sore and hot
Hamamelis	In cold	In warm air	Profuse bleeding with tightness in bridge of nose
Millefolium	Application of cold on bridge of nose	After violent exertion	Stuffed-up nose
Phosphorus	In open air and after sleep	With physical or mental exertion	Handkerchief often bloody
Pulsatilla	In open air	In warm room	Coryza, stoppage of right nostril, loss of smell

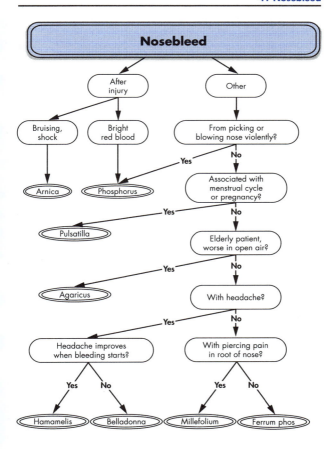

42 Period pains

- When the appropriate medicine has been established and is effective for the acute symptoms, it may be possible to use the same medicine bd for days 12–18 of the cycle to prevent the symptoms or reduce the severity.

Homeopathic medicine	Better	Worse	Other
Actaea rac (aka Cimicifuga)	Warmth and eating	In the morning	Pelvic pain, amenorrhoea
Belladonna	Sitting up	Touch and lying down	Throbbing pain radiating from nipples, breasts feel heavy
Borax	Evening and cold weather	Warm weather	Menses profuse, nausea and pain in stomach extending into small of back
Caulophyllum	Warmth	Motion	Spasmodic and severe pains over abdomen. Dysmenorrhoea
Chamomilla	Pressure	Touch and in morning	Patient complains of general pain, inflamed nipples tender to touch
Mag phos	Warmth	In the cold and at night	Colic and irregularities of cycle
Pulsatilla	Open air and motion	Heat	Amenorrhoea, nausea and downward pressure. Painful flow. Diarrhoea possible
Sepia	Exercise and warmth of bed	In cold air	Flatulence with headache, sickness in the morning, painful vagina

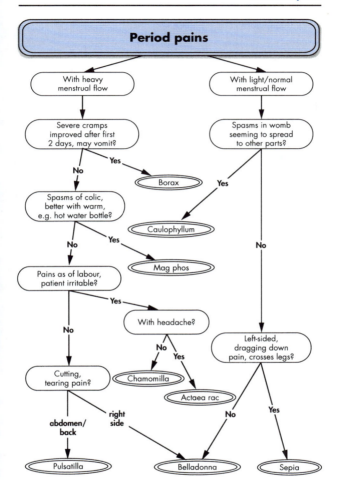

43 Perspiration

- Distinction should be made between general excessive perspiration and fever.
- Importance of increased fluid intake should be stressed.

Homeopathic medicine	Better	Worse	Other
Acid fluor	Cold while walking	Warmth in the morning	Profuse, sour offensive perspiration, often inflammation of finger joints
Alumina	In open air and from cold washing	In the afternoon and in warm room	Chapped and dry skin, brittle nails
Amyl nit	Cool air	Anxiety	Flushed face and chest pains. Bursting headache
Calc carb	In dry weather	Physical or mental exertion	Rheumatoid pains in extremities
Lycopodium	Motion and warm drinks	Heat or warm room	Abscesses beneath skin, hives and violent itching. Varicose veins
Merc sol	In cool	Warmth of bed and at night	Excessive odorous perspiration, itching skin
Silica	Warmth	In the morning	Abscesses and boils on skin. Sciatica. Cold sweat on hands and feet
Sulphur	Dry warm weather	Scratching and washing	Dry, scaly unhealthy skin with itching and burning. Patient feels hot

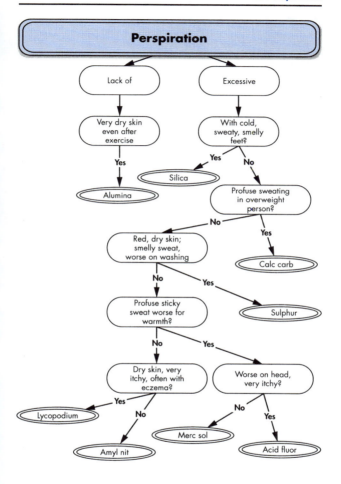

Perspiration

Lack of → Very dry skin even after exercise → **Yes** → Alumina

Excessive → With cold, sweaty, smelly feet?
- **Yes** → Silica
- **No** → Profuse sweating in overweight person?
  - **Yes** → Calc carb
  - **No** → Red, dry skin; smelly sweat, worse on washing
    - **Yes** → Sulphur
    - **No** → Profuse sticky sweat worse for warmth?
      - **Yes** → Worse on head, very itchy?
        - **Yes** → Acid fluor
        - **No** → Merc sol
      - **No** → Dry skin, very itchy, often with eczema?
        - **Yes** → Lycopodium
        - **No** → Amyl nit

44 Pre-menstrual syndrome

- **FIM** – choice between Pulsatilla and Sepia.
- Pulsatilla more successful in fair-skinned and affectionate women with a tendency to be weepy; Sepia in tall slim women with dark complexion.

Homeopathic medicine	Better	Worse	Other
Calc carb	In dry climate and lying down	Mental or physical exertion and cold	Headache, colic and chilliness. Cold, damp feet
Lachesis	Warm applications	Pressure of clothes and after sleep	Breasts inflamed, flashes of heat, headache and fainting spells
Lilium tig	Fresh air	In warm room	Pain down thighs. Pruritus
Lycopodium	Motion and being uncovered	Any form of heat	Pain in right ovarian region. Burning sensation in vagina
Nat mur	In the open air and pressure against back	Lying down	Irregular periods, usually profuse flow
Nux vom	Sleep and strong pressure	In the morning and after mental exertion	Irregular cycle
Pulsatilla	Open air and from motion	Heat and a warm room	Amenorrhoea. Chilliness, nausea and downward pressure. Sometimes associated with diarrhoea
Sepia	Exercise. Pressure and warmth of bed	In morning and evening	Period often late, sickness in the morning and vagina may be painful

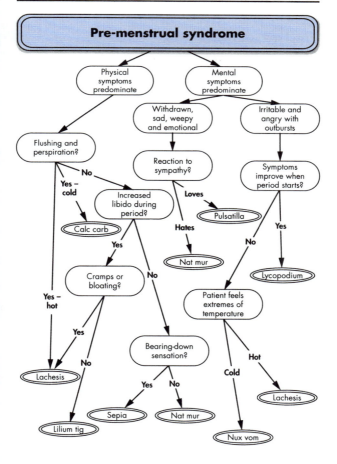

Pre-menstrual syndrome

45 Rheumatic and arthritic pain

- **FIM** – Rhus tox if better for movement, Bryonia if better for rest.
- Rhus Tox/Ruta 5% gel useful topically in many cases.
- See also Chart 50, Sports injuries and Chart 51, Sprains and strains.

Homeopathic medicine	Better	Worse	Other
Apis	In open air and after cold bathing	Heat and touch	Oedema, synovitis. Swollen knee. Rheumatic pain in back and limbs. Sore sensitive skin
Bryonia	Application of cold	Warmth and motion	Knees stiff and painful. Joints red, swollen and hot
Causticum	Warmth, especially heat of bed	Dry, cold winds	Weak ankles and dull pain in arms and hands
Dulcamara	Movement	At night	Pain in shin bones. Often associated with skin eruptions
Kalmia	Warmth	Motion	Pains affect hips to knees and feet. Sense of coldness in limbs. Joints red, hot and swollen
Ledum	Cold	At night and from heat of bed	Pains in foot and in joints, especially small joints. Swollen, hot. Throbbing in right shoulder
Rhododendron	With warmth and eating	At rest and at night. Extreme sensitivity to changes in weather	Swollen joints, inflammation of big toe joint. Pain especially on right side of limbs. Stiff neck
Rhus tox	With movement and in warmth	In the cold and at night	Rheumatic pains over neck, thighs and extremities

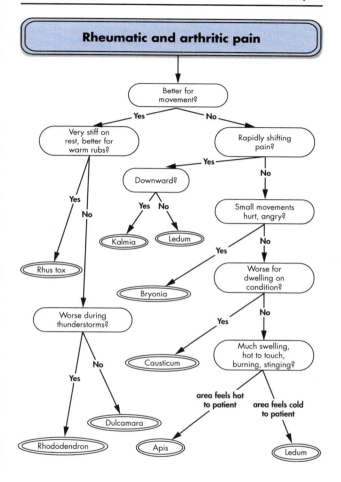

Rheumatic and arthritic pain

Better for movement?

Yes — Very stiff on rest, better for warm rubs?

No — Rapidly shifting pain?

Yes (Rapidly shifting pain?) — Downward?
  - Yes → Kalmia
  - No → Ledum

No (Rapidly shifting pain?) — Small movements hurt, angry?
  - Yes → Bryonia
  - No → Worse for dwelling on condition?
    - Yes → Causticum
    - No → Much swelling, hot to touch, burning, stinging?
      - area feels hot to patient → Apis
      - area feels cold to patient → Ledum

Very stiff on rest, better for warm rubs?
  - Yes → Rhus tox
  - No → Worse during thunderstorms?
    - Yes → Rhododendron
    - No → Dulcamara

46 Sciatica

- This is a very changeable condition – the same patient may present different symptoms with each episode and may require different medicines each time.

Homeopathic medicine	Better	Worse	Other
Ammon mur	Lying down	Sitting down	Shooting and tearing pain. Often associated with backache and sweaty feet
Bryonia	Cold	With warmth and motion	Painful stiffness in neck and back, knees stiff and painful
Carbo sulph	In open air	In warm	Pains in lower limbs with cramps. Fingers swollen
Colocynth	Pressure and heat	Gentle touch	Pain from hip to knee. Stiffness of joint. Sciatica particularly on left side
Gelsemium	In open air and continued motion	In damp weather	Fatigue after slight exercise. Trembling in limbs
Gnaphalium	Sitting and flexing limbs	At night and with motion	Cramps in calves of legs and feet when in bed. Pain in joints and back
Lycopodium	Warm food and drink	On right side	Numbness in limbs, especially while at rest and at night. Feet sweaty
Mag phos	In the warm and with pressure	In cold and at night	General muscular weakness and feet very tender
Rhus tox	In the warm	During sleep and cold	May be associated with hot, painful swelling of joints and tingling in feet

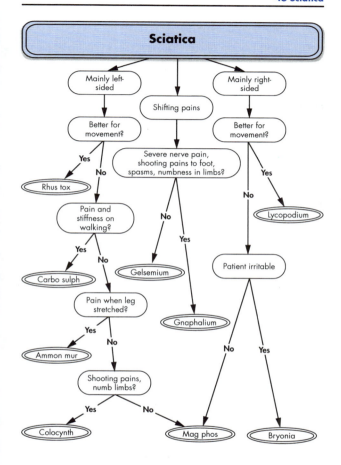

47 Sleep problems

- **FIM** – Avena sat, Coffea and Passiflora either alone or in combination may be useful.
- For persistent insomnia, a constitutional medicine may be more suitable – a detailed consultation would be required. Consider referral.
- Conventional medication should be continued unless stopped by the prescribing doctor.

Homeopathic medicine	Better	Worse	Other
Argent nit	Fresh air and cold	Warmth and at menstrual period	Cannot fall asleep due to imagination. Dreams featuring snakes
Arsen alb	Heat and warm drinks	In wet weather and cold drinks	Disturbed, anxious and restless. Requires head to be raised with pillows. May sleep with hands over head
Avena sat	None recorded	None recorded	Sleeplessness may be associated with alcoholism or drug addiction
Belladonna	In quiet and moderate temperatures	Touch and noise	Restless, screams out in sleep. Often sleeps with hands under head
Chamomilla	Being carried (children). Warm and wet weather	Heat and emotional upset	May cry out during sleep, anxious and frightened dreams
Coffea	Lying down and holding ice in the mouth	Emotional upset	Wakes up very early with a start. Sleep disturbed by dreams
Equisetum	Lying down	Movement	Enuresis
Nux vom	Following rest	After eating spices	Broken sleep, dreams associated with urgency
Passiflora	Peace and quiet	Mental worries and exhaustion	Restless and nocturnal cough
Phosphorus	Cold food and washing with cold water	Physical or mental exertion and warm food and drink	Drowsiness after meals. Goes to sleep late

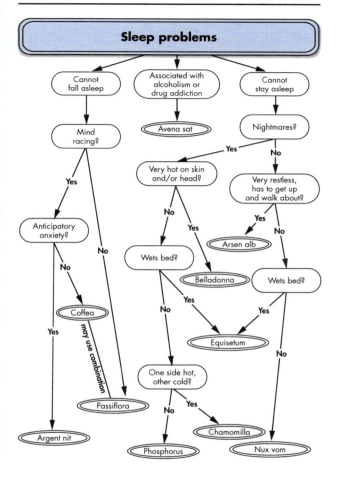

48 Smoking

- Homeopathy can be effective alone but often works best complementary to a directed NRT (nicotine replacement therapy) programme.
- Nux vom should be taken in the 200c potency twice daily from day of stopping for 5–10 days.
- Nux vom pre-eminently the medicine for many of the conditions found in modern life.
- To alleviate acute cravings, use Staphisagria or Caladium at a dose of 30c qds.

Homeopathic medicine	Better	Worse	Other
Caladium	After sleeping	Warm air	Headaches following smoking. Belching
Nux vom	Rest	Touch and if other ailments present. Mental exertion	Stress of modern life, irritability, digestive disturbances. Sleep problems
Staphisagria	Rest	After emotional upset	Headache with yawning, craving for tobacco. Nausea, diarrhoea

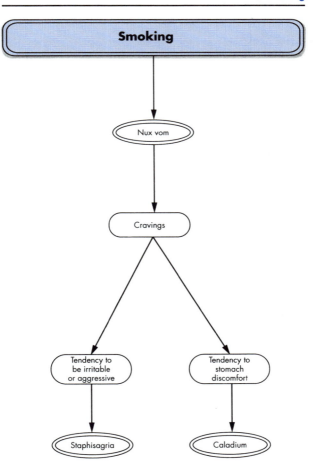

49 Sore throat

- **FIM** – Belladonna where fever, red, hot, sore to swallow, especially in children.
- Hypericum/Calendula tincture useful as a gargle – 5 drops in water.
- If appropriate, herbal Echinacea can be very valuable to boost the immune system – 825 mg daily (adult dose).

Homeopathic medicine	Better	Worse	Other
Aconite	In open air	In warm room	Red and dry with swollen tonsils
Baryta carb	Walking in open air	Heat	Difficulty swallowing. May be associated with overuse of voice
Belladonna	Cold drinks	Heat	Dry throat, enlarged tonsils. Throat feels constricted. Red and hot
Gelsemium	In the open air	After emotional upset	Difficulty swallowing warm food, throat feels rough and burning. Ear may also be affected
Hepar sulph	After eating and in damp weather	Dry, cold winds and cool air	Gums and mouth painful to touch and bleed readily
Merc sol	Sucking ice cubes	At night and from warm room and warm bed	Raw and burning throat with loss of voice. Ulcerated. Excessive saliva
Phosphorus	Cool open air and cold food	After physical and mental exertion and from warm food and drink	Thirst for very cold water. Bleeding gums
Phytolacca	Warm dry weather	In cold weather	Dark-red or bluish sore throat. Sensation of lump in throat

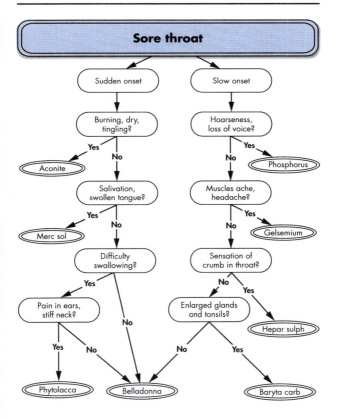

50 Sports injuries

- Arnica 5% gel useful topically in most cases for bruising.
- Ruta/Rhus tox 5% gel used topically for sprains and strains.
- See also Chart 51, Sprains and strains.

Homeopathic medicine	Better	Worse	Other
Aconite	Open air	Warm room	Inflamed joints, knee problems and fear and anxiety
Arnica	Lying down	Least touch	Injuries involving bruising. Physical and mental exhaustion
Bellis perennis	In cool	After hot bath and warmth of bed	Injuries to breast and trauma of pelvic area. Good medicine for sprains and bruises
Bryonia	With pressure and rest	Warmth and motion	Knees stiff and painful. Pain in neck
Hypericum	After rubbing and lying quietly	In cold and with touch	Pain in toes and fingers especially the tips. Pain in shoulders
Ledum	At night and from heat of bed	Cold	Ankle sprain and shoulder injuries, especially right shoulder
Nat sulph	In dry weather and changing position	In damp	Pain in hip joint, stiffness of knees. Pains in back of neck
Phosphorus	Cold food and in the open air. Washing with cold water	Touch, warm food or drink	Burning in the back. Pain in elbow and shoulder joints. Dry tickly cough
Symphytum	Rest	Activity	Any injury with bone involvement

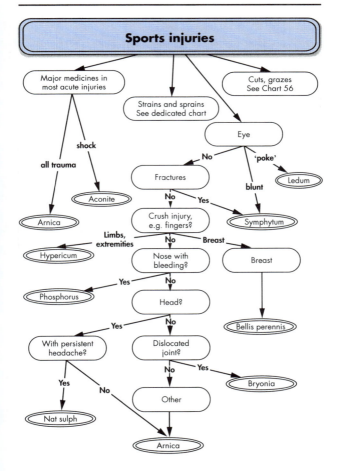

51 Sprains and strains

- Rhus Tox/Ruta 5% gel or Arnica 5% gel as appropriate useful topically in most cases.

Homeopathic medicine	Better	Worse	Other
Apis	Uncovered and with application of cold	Heat and touch	Oedema in extremities, synovitis
Arnica	Lying down	Least touch and motion	Effects of mental and physical exertion. Used for traumatic injuries
Bellis perennis	Motion	Warmth of bed	Used for sprains and bruises, injuries to breast
Bryonia	Rest	Motion	Patient usually irritable and thirsty
Rhus tox	Application of heat. Initial movement worse, subsequent movement much easier. Stretching limbs	Cold	Skin often red, swollen and intense itching
Ruta grav	Warmth and gentle rubbing	Lying down and cold	Used for muscular sprains. Also used for eye strain

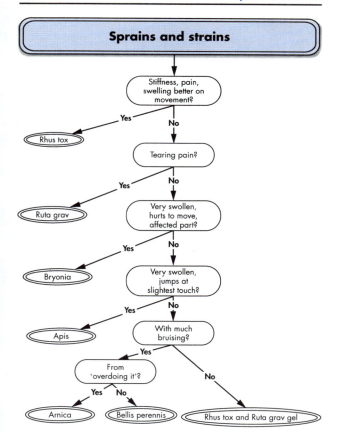

52 Teething

- **FIM** – Chamomilla.

Homeopathic medicine	Better	Worse	Other
Belladonna	With light covering	Touch and lying down	Skin dry and hot, possible high feverish state
Borax	Late evening	Warm weather	Baby cries while being nursed. Mouth hot and tender
Calc phos	In summer	Cold weather	Associated with swollen tonsils. Teeth develop slowly
Chamomilla	Being carried	Warm food or drink	Restless, needs constant attention
Merc sol	In moderate temperature	At night	Severe pain on touch and from chewing
Nux vom	In the evening and while at rest	In the morning after eating	Often associated with small aphthous ulcers, swollen gums

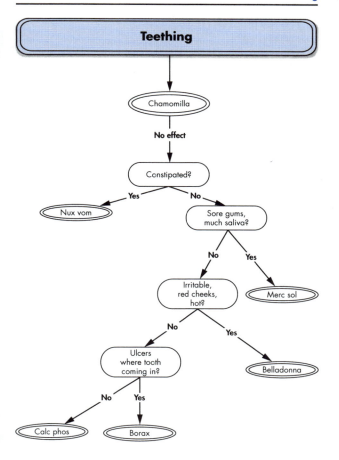

Teething

Chamomilla

No effect

Constipated?

Yes → Nux vom

No → Sore gums, much saliva?

No → Irritable, red cheeks, hot?

Yes → Merc sol

No → Ulcers where tooth coming in?

Yes → Belladonna

No → Calc phos

Yes → Borax

53 Travel sickness

- Acupressure wrist bands are effective in some cases.
- Appropriate medicine should be given in the 30c potency 1 hour before journey, on departure and every 2 hours during journey if necessary, up to a maximum of six doses in 24 hours.
- If no single medicine is strongly indicated, the most appropriate two medicines may be alternated, up to a maximum of six total doses in 24 hours.
- See Chart 4, Anxiety and shock for medicines associated with anxiety about travel.

Homeopathic medicine	Better	Worse	Other
Argent nit	Cool air	Emotion and warmth	Belching, nausea and vomiting, wind. Anxiety about journey
Borax	In cool weather	Noise and tobacco smoke	Nervous and sensitive to sudden noises. Abdominal distension
Cocculus	Cool air	With eating and after loss of sleep and emotional disturbance	Nausea from travelling in cars and boats. Hiccoughs and spasmodic yawning
Coffea	Warmth, lying down and holding ice in the mouth	Open air	Irritability
Nux vom	After sleeping	Eating, especially spicy food	Sour taste in mouth, much retching; constipation
Petroleum	Warm air	Dampness	Heartburn and belching, hunger. Car motion
Tabacum	In fresh air and with eyes closed	Extremes of heat and cold	Nausea, worse with smell of tobacco smoke. Vomiting on least motion. Sea sickness

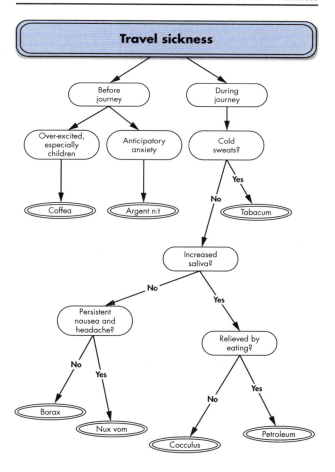

Travel sickness

Before journey
- Over-excited, especially children → Coffea
- Anticipatory anxiety → Argent nit

During journey
- Cold sweats?
  - Yes → Tabacum
  - No → Increased saliva?
    - No → Persistent nausea and headache?
      - No → Borax
      - Yes → Nux vom
    - Yes → Relieved by eating?
      - No → Cocculus
      - Yes → Petroleum

54 Urinary problems (acute)

- **FIM** – Causticum if increased frequency, Cantharis if pain/burning mainly on urination.
- Sabal serr mother tincture or tincture can be useful taken at night – 3–5 drops in water for men with increased urinary frequency.

Homeopathic medicine	Better	Worse	Other
Acid nit	Movement	In evening and at night	Scanty urine, dark in colour. Burning and stinging sensation
Argent nit	In fresh air and cold	In warmth and at night	Burning pain and itching. Divided stream of urine
Baryta carb	Walking in open air	In warm atmosphere	Frequent urge to urinate
Cantharis	Warmth	Drinking cold water	Scalding urine passes drop-wise. Constant desire to urinate
Causticum	In warmth and heat of bed	Cold air and movement	Involuntary passage of urine when coughing, sneezing or excited
Lycopodium	Being uncovered	Heat or warm room	Pain in back before urinating ceases after flow. Much straining. Polyuria during the night. Male impotence
Nux vom	In the evening at rest	In the morning and in the cold	Irritable bladder, frequent passage of small quantities of urine
Sabal serr	After sleep	In the cold	Constant desire to urinate. Enuresis
Sarsasparilla	In cool dry air	At night and after urinating	Urine dribbles, bladder distended and tender. Child often screams before and while passing urine
Silica	Exercise and warmth of bed	Cold air	Chronic cystitis. Bearing-down sensation
Staphisagria	Warmth and rest at night	Emotional upset and tobacco. Women – after sexual activity	Burning sensation during urination. May be associated with prostatic trouble

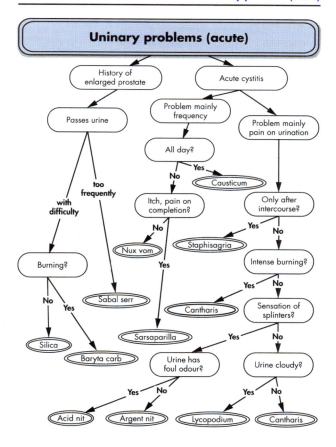

Urinary problems (acute)

- History of enlarged prostate
  - Passes urine
    - **with difficulty**
      - Burning?
        - No → Silica
        - Yes → Baryta carb
    - **too frequently**
      - Sabal serr

- Acute cystitis
  - Problem mainly frequency
    - All day?
      - Yes → Causticum
      - No → Itch, pain on completion?
        - No → Nux vom
        - Yes → Sarsaparilla
  - Problem mainly pain on urination
    - Only after intercourse?
      - Yes → Staphisagria
      - No → Intense burning?
        - Yes → Cantharis
        - No → Sensation of splinters?
          - Yes → Urine has foul odour?
            - Yes → Acid nit
            - No → Argent nit
          - No → Urine cloudy?
            - Yes → Lycopodium
            - No → Cantharis

55 Warts and verrucae

- **FIM** for all conditions – Thuja 30c, twice daily.
- Thuja tincture or 5% ointment also useful topically.
- Topical and oral treatment may be used concurrently.
- Treatment may take 4–16 weeks.

Homeopathic medicine	Better	Worse	Other
Acid nit	Mild weather and warm covering	At night and in extremes of temperature	Large jagged warts that bleed on washing
Ant crud	Warm bath	Aggravated by heat and cold bathing	Dry, scaly skin often with pustular eruptions
Causticum	Not recorded	Not recorded	Large jagged warts, especially on fingers and nose
Sabina	Cool, fresh air	Heat	Warts that itch and burn
Thuja	None recorded	After scratching	A variety of skin eruptions (including verrucae), and nail problems

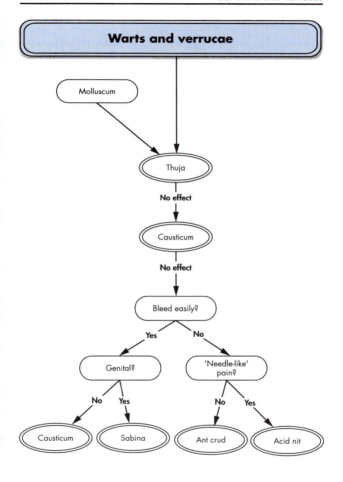

Warts and verrucae

Molluscum

Thuja

No effect

Causticum

No effect

Bleed easily?

Yes — Genital?

No — Causticum

Yes — Sabina

No — 'Needle-like' pain?

No — Ant crud

Yes — Acid nit

56 Wounds

- For superficial cuts and grazes, clean wound with diluted Calendula or Hypericum/Calendula tincture then use the 5% cream or ointment (latter better as greasy base seals wound). **Do not use topical products on deep wounds**.
- Superficial wounds may be also dressed with tea tree preparations; however, this herbal product does cause an allergic response in some patients.
- Oral and topical treatment may be used concurrently.

Homeopathic medicine	Better	Worse	Other
Calendula	Warmth	In the evening	Superficial burns and scalds
Hepar sulph	Wrapping up affected parts	Cool air	Used to treat ulcers and cold sores. Also abscesses, chapped skin and where infection present
Hypericum	Lying quietly	Application of pressure. Motion	Blood and crush injuries. Shock
Ledum	Cold	At night and from heat of bed	Puncture wounds. May be indicated if patient suffers from eczema
Silica	Warmth	Cold	Promotes expulsion of foreign bodies from tissues. May be indicated where injury suppurating

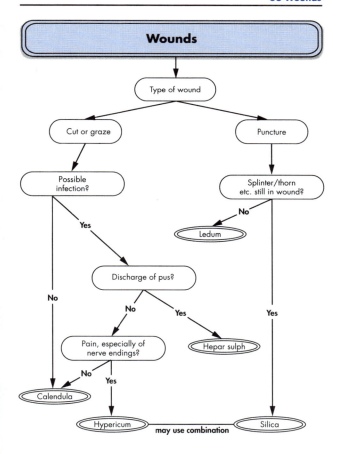

Appendix 1

Useful addresses

Organisations supporting prescribers

European Committee for Homeopathy (ECH) Secretariat
Chaussee de Bruxelles 132, Box 1
1190 Brussels
Belgium
Tel: +32 2 345 3597
E-mail: info@homeopathyeurope.org
Website: www.homeopathyeurope.org

The Faculty of Homeopathy
Hahnemann House
29 Park Street West
Luton LU1 3BE
Tel: +44 (0)870 444 3950
Fax: +44 (0)870 444 3960
Website: www.trusthomeopathy.org

The Faculty of Homeopathy in Scotland
Glasgow Homeopathic Hospital
1053 Great Western Road
Glasgow G12 0XQ
Tel: +44 (0)141 211 1617
Fax: +44 (0)141 211 1610
E-mail: hom-inform@dial.pipex.com

The Society of Homeopaths
11 Brookfield
Duncan Close
Moulton Park
Northampton NN3 6 WL
Tel: +44 (0)845 450 6611
Fax: +44 (0)845 450 6622
Website: www.homeopathy-soh.org

British Holistic Medical Association
39 Lansdown Place
Hove
East Sussex BN3 1EL

Tel: +44 (0)1273 725951
Website: www.bhma.org

British Institute of Homeopathy
Endeavour House
80 High Street
Egham
Surrey TW20 9HE
Tel: +44 (0)1784 473800
E-mail: info@the-hma.org
Website: www.britinsthom.com

United Kingdom Homoeopathic Medical Association (UKHMA)
6 Livingstone Road
Gravesend
Kent DA12 5DZ
Tel/fax: +44 (0)1474 560336
Website: www.homoeopathy.org/

More information

Hom-Inform and British Homoeopathic Library
Glasgow Homeopathic Hospital
1053 Great Western Road
Glasgow G12 0XQ
Tel: +44 (0)141 211 1617
Fax: +44 (0)141 211 1610
E-mail: hom-inform@dial.pipex.com

The Prince of Wales Foundation for Integrated Health
12 Chillingworth Road
London N7 8QJ
Tel: +44 (0)20 7619 5140
Website: www.fihealth.org.uk

BHA Book Service
20 Main Street
Busby
Glasgow G76 8DU
Tel: +44 (0)845 225 5492
Website: www.bhabooks.com

Patients' associations

British Homeopathic Association
Hahnemann House
29 Park Street West
Luton LU1 3BE
Tel: +44 (0)870 444 3950

Fax: +44 (0)870 444 3960
Website: www.trusthomeopathy.org

The Patients' Association for Anthroposophical Medicine
St Luke's Medical Centre
51 Cairns Cross Road
Stroud
Glos GL4 4EX

Hospitals

Bristol Homeopathic Hospital
Cotham Hill
Cotham
Bristol BS6 6JU
Tel: +44 (0)117 973 1231
Website: www.ubht.nhs.uk/homeopathy/

Liverpool Homeopathic Hospital
Department of Homeopathic Medicine
Mossley Hill Hospital
Park Avenue
Liverpool L18 8BU
Tel: +44 (0)151 285 3707

Glasgow Homeopathic Hospital
1053 Great Western Road
Glasgow G12 0XQ
Tel: +44 (0)141 337 1824
Fax: +44 (0)141 211 1610
Website: ghh.info/welcome.htm

Royal London Homoeopathic Hospital
Great Ormond Street
London WC1 N 3HR
Tel: +44 (0)845 155 5000 (Patient services: +44 (0)20 7391 8888)
Website: www.uclh.nhs.uk/rlhh

Tunbridge Wells Homoeopathic Hospital
Church Road
Tunbridge Wells
Kent TN1 1JU
Tel: +44 (0)1892 542977

Clinic not NHS, but a registered charity

Manchester Homoeopathic Clinic
Brunswick Street
Ardwick
Manchester M13 9ST
Tel: +44 (0)161 273 2446

UK suppliers of homeopathic medicines

Ainsworths Homeopathic Pharmacy
36 New Cavendish Street
London W1G 8UF
Tel: +44 (0)20 7935 5330
Fax: +44 (0)20 7486 4313
Website: www.ainsworths.com
(also supply books and homeopathic veterinary products)

Freeman's Homeopathic Pharmacy
18–20 Main Street
Busby
Glasgow G76 8DU
Tel: +44 (0)141 644 1165/+44 (0)845 225 5155
Fax: +44 (0)141 644 5735/+44 (0)845 225 5255
Website: www.freemans.uk.com
(also supply books and homeopathic veterinary products)

Helios Homoeopathy
89–97 Camden Road
Tunbridge Wells
Kent TN1 2QR
Tel: +44 (0)1892 537254
Fax: +44 (0)1892 546850
Website: www.helios.co.uk
(also supply books and veterinary products)

Nelsonbach
Broadheath House
83 Parkside
Wimbledon
London SW19 5LP
Tel: +44 (0)20 8780 4200
Fax: +44 (0)20 8780 5871
Website: www.nelsonbach.com

New Era Laboratories, Seven Seas Ltd
Hedon Road
Marfleet
Hull HU9 5NJ
Tel: +44 (0)1482 375234
Fax: +44 (0)1482 374345
Website: www.seven-seas.ltd.uk

Weleda UK
Heanor Road
Ilkeston
Derbyshire DE7 8DR
Tel: +44 (0)115 944 8200
Fax: +44 (0)115 944 8210
Website: www.weleda.co.uk

Appendix 2

Further information

Training in homeopathy

Information on UK postgraduate and undergraduate degrees in complementary and alternative medicine including homeopathy may be found at www.rccm.org.uk/static/Links_Courses.aspx?m=7

A comprehensive and current listing of colleges around the world may be found online at the Homeopathy Home Page (www.homeopathyhome. com).

Training is also offered in the UK and overseas by the Faculty of Homeopathy (see above) and in the UK by Continuing Professional Education Centres (e.g. National Health Service Education for Scotland).

Online sources of information

Alternative Medicine Foundation
www.amfoundation.org/homeopathinfo.htm

British Homeopathic Library
www.hom-inform.org/

Elixirs.com – theory and practice newsletters
www.elixirs.com/newsletter.htm

Homeopathic education services
www.homeopathic.com/

Homeopathic internet resources
www.holisticmed.com/www/homeopathy.html

Kent Homeopathic Associates
www.repertory.org/links.html

Links
www.homeoint.org/lienamis.htm#english

Homeopathyhome – general resource
www.homeopathyhome.com/reference/index.shtml

Homeoweb – general resource
www2.antenna.nl/homeoweb/

National Electronic Library for Health: Complementary and Alternative Medicine Specialist Library: Homeopathy
www.library.nhs.uk/cam/SearchResults.aspx?tabID=288&catID=9652

United States National Center for Complementary and Alternative Medicine (NCCAM)
www.nccam.nih.gov

Further reading

Family guides

Gemmell D (1997). *Everyday Homeopathy*. Beaconsfield: Beaconsfield Publishers.

Gibson D (2005). *First Aid Homoeopathy in Accidents & Ailments*, 18th edn. Glasgow: BHA Book Service.

Hunter F, Kayne S (1997). *People are Pets*. Glasgow: BHA Book Service (Human & Veterinary).

Lockie A (1998). *Family Guide to Homeopathy*. London: Penguin Books (Hamish Hamilton).

General reading

Handley R (1997). *In Search of the Later Hahnemann*. Beaconsfield: Beaconsfield Publishers.

Wright-Hubbard E (1990). *Homeopathy as Art and Science*. Beaconsfield: Beaconsfield Publishers.

Wood M (1992). *The Magical Staff. The Vitalist Tradition in Western Medicine*. Berkeley, CA: North Atlantic Books.

Practice of homeopathy

Swayne J (1997). *Homeopathic Method*. Oxford: Elsevier (Churchill Livingstone).

Swayne J (2000). *International Dictionary of Homeopathy*. Oxford: Elsevier (Churchill Livingstone).

Watson I (2004). *Guide to the Methodologies of Homeopathy*. Kendal: Cutting Edge Books.

Materia medicas and repertories

Boericke W (2005). *Homoeopathic Materia Medica with Repertory*, 2nd British edn, 5th impression. Sittingbourne: Homoeopathic Book Service (various editions available).

Clarke J H (1952). *The Prescriber*, 9th edn. London: Random House Books (CW Danie).

Clarke J (1991). *Dictionary of Practical Materia Medica*. London: Random House Books (CW Danie).

Kent J T (1993). *Repertory of the Homeopathic Materia Medica*. Sittingbourne: Homeopathic Book Service.

Kent J T (2000). *Materia Medica of Homeopathic Remedies*. Sittingbourne: Homeopathic Book Service.

Murphy R (2003). *Homeopathic Remedy Guide*, 2nd edn. Virginia: Lotus Health Institute.

Murphy R (2005). *Homeopathic Clinical Repertory*, 3rd edn. Virginia: Lotus Health Institute.

Phatak S R (1988). *Phatak's Materia Medica of Homoeopathic Medicines*. London: Foxlee-Vaughan.

Schroyens F (2004). *Synthesis*, 9th edn. London: Homeopathic Book Publishers.

Vermeulen F (2000). *Concordant Materia Medica*. Haarlem, NL: Emryss Publishers.

Mother and children

Castro M (1992). *Homoeopathy for Mother and Baby*. London: Macmillan.

Pinto G, Feldman M (2000). *Homeopathy for Children*. London: Random House Books (CW Danie).

Webb P (1999). *Homoeopathy for Midwives (and All Pregnant Women)*. Glasgow: BHA Book Service.

Research topics

Bellavite P, Signorini A (1995). *Homeopathy. A Frontier in Medical Science*. Berkeley, CA: North Atlantic Books.

Dean M E (2004). *The Trials of Homeopathy*. Stuttgart: KVC Verlag.

Sport

Thomas E (2000). *Homeopathy for Sport, Exercise and Dance*. Beaconsfield: Beaconsfield Publishers.

Theory of homeopathy

Boyd H (1989). *Introduction to Homeopathic Medicine*. Beaconsfield: Beaconsfield Publishers.

Lessell C (2003). *Companion to Homeopathic Studies*. London: Random House Books (CW Danie).

Travel

Lessell C (1999). *World Travellers' Manual of Homeopathy*. London: Random House Books (CW Danie).

Pharmacy

Kayne S (2001). *Complementary Therapies for Pharmacists*. London: Pharmaceutical Press.

Kayne S (2006). *Homeopathic Pharmacy*, 2nd edn. Edinburgh: Churchill Livingstone.

Veterinary

Saxton J and Gregory P (2005). *Textbook of Veterinary Homeopathy*. Beaconsfield: Beaconsfield Publishers.

Hunter F (2004). *Everyday Homeopathy for Animals*. Beaconsfield: Beaconsfield Publishers.

Flower remedies and tissue salts

Chancellor P (2005). *Illustrated Handbook of Bach Flower Remedies*. London: Random House Books (Vermillion).

Boericke W and Dewey W (2003). *Schüssler's Twelve Tissue Remedies*. Sittingbourne: Homoeopathic Book Service.

Appendix 3

Materia medica

This materia medica reflects the recommended usage of medicines in this book – all the medicines have many other homeopathic applications. Further, it includes only the applications indicated in the prescribing charts. Some other applications may be found on the supplementary page facing each chart.

Remedy	Ailment
Acid fluor	Perspiration
Acid nit	Breastfeeding
Acid nit	Haemorrhoids
Acid nit	Mouth problems
Acid nit	Urinary problems (acute)
Acid nit	Warts and verrucae
Acid phos	Bereavement
Acid phos	Diarrhoea
Acid phos	Fatigue (acute)
Acid pic	Fatigue (acute)
Acid sal	Ear problems
Aconite	Anxiety and shock
Aconite	Burns
Aconite	Cold and flu
Aconite	Cough
Aconite	Ear problems
Aconite	Fever
Aconite	Injury
Aconite	Labour
Aconite	Sore throat

Aconite	Sports injuries
Actaea rac	Backache
Actaea rac	Menopause
Actaea rac	Period pains
Aesculus	Haemorrhoids
Agaricus	Itch
Agaricus	Nosebleed
Ailanthus	Glandular fever
Aletris	Morning sickness
Allium cepa	Cold and flu
Allium cepa	Hay fever
Aloe soc	Diarrhoea
Aloe soc	Haemorrhoids
Alumina	Constipation
Alumina	Perspiration
Ambrosia	Hay fever
Ammon mur	Hay fever
Ammon mur	Sciatica
Amygdalus per	Morning sickness
Amyl nit	Hot flushes
Amyl nit	Perspiration
Anacardium	Nausea and vomiting
Ant crud	Chickenpox and shingles
Ant crud	Nausea and vomiting
Ant crud	Warts and verrucae
Ant tart	Backache
Ant tart	Chickenpox and shingles
Ant tart	Cough
Apis	Abscesses and boils
Apis	Bites and stings
Apis	Chickenpox and shingles
Apis	Ear problems

Apis	Itch
Apis	Rheumatic and arthritic pain
Apis	Sprains and strains
Apomorphinum	Morning sickness
Argent nit	Anxiety and shock
Argent nit	Bedwetting
Argent nit	Cramp
Argent nit	Diarrhoea
Argent nit	Eye problems
Argent nit	Flatulence
Argent nit	Sleep problems
Argent nit	Travel sickness
Argent nit	Urinary problems (acute)
Arnica	Anxiety and shock
Arnica	Backache
Arnica	Bruising
Arnica	Cramp
Arnica	Eye problems
Arnica	Fatigue (acute)
Arnica	Gout
Arnica	Injury
Arnica	Labour
Arnica	Menopause
Arnica	Nosebleed
Arnica	Sports injuries
Arnica	Sprains and strains
Arsen alb	Anxiety and shock
Arsen alb	Bedwetting
Arsen alb	Bereavement
Arsen alb	Chickenpox and shingles
Arsen alb	Cold sores
Arsen alb	Diarrhoea

Arsen alb	Eczema and dermatitis
Arsen alb	Fever
Arsen alb	Nausea and vomiting
Arsen alb	Sleep problems
Arsen iod	Catarrh and sinus problems
Arsen iod	Cold and flu
Arundo	Hay fever
Aurum met	Hot flushes
Avena sat	Sleep problems
Baptisia	Fever
Baryta carb	Haemorrhoids
Baryta carb	Sore throat
Baryta carb	Urinary problems (acute)
Belladonna	Abscesses and boils
Belladonna	Acne
Belladonna	Bedwetting
Belladonna	Breastfeeding
Belladonna	Burns
Belladonna	Cold and flu
Belladonna	Colic
Belladonna	Cough
Belladonna	Ear problems
Belladonna	Fever
Belladonna	Flatulence
Belladonna	Glandular fever
Belladonna	Gout
Belladonna	Headache and migraine
Belladonna	Hot flushes
Belladonna	Mouth problems
Belladonna	Nosebleed
Belladonna	Period pains
Belladonna	Sleep problems

Belladonna	Sore throat
Belladonna	Teething
Bellis perennis	Bruising
Bellis perennis	Labour
Bellis perennis	Sports injuries
Bellis perennis	Sprains and strains
Borax	Breastfeeding
Borax	Mouth problems
Borax	Period pains
Borax	Teething
Borax	Travel sickness
Bryonia	Backache
Bryonia	Breastfeeding
Bryonia	Cold and flu
Bryonia	Cough
Bryonia	Cramp
Bryonia	Fever
Bryonia	Headache and migraine
Bryonia	Mouth problems
Bryonia	Rheumatic and arthritic pain
Bryonia	Sciatica
Bryonia	Sports injuries
Bryonia	Sprains and strains
Caladium	Smoking
Calc carb	Perspiration
Calc carb	Pre-menstrual syndrome
Calc phos	Teething
Calendula	Wounds
Cantharis	Bites and stings
Cantharis	Burns
Cantharis	Urinary problems (acute)
Capsicum	Cold sores

Carbo sulph	Ear problems
Carbo sulph	Sciatica
Carbo veg	Colic
Carbo veg	Flatulence
Caulophyllum	Labour
Caulophyllum	Menopause
Caulophyllum	Period pains
Causticum	Bedwetting
Causticum	Burns
Causticum	Chickenpox and shingles
Causticum	Haemorrhoids
Causticum	Rheumatic and arthritic pain
Causticum	Urinary problems (acute)
Causticum	Warts and verrucae
Chamomilla	Breastfeeding
Chamomilla	Colic
Chamomilla	Cramp
Chamomilla	Diarrhoea
Chamomilla	Ear problems
Chamomilla	Labour
Chamomilla	Period pains
Chamomilla	Sleep problems
Chamomilla	Teething
China	Ear problems
China	Fatigue (acute)
Cinnabaris	Catarrh and sinus problems
Cistus can	Glandular fever
Cocculus	Fatigue (acute)
Cocculus	Morning sickness
Cocculus	Travel sickness
Coffea	Sleep problems
Coffea	Travel sickness

Colchicum	Gout
Collinsonia	Haemorrhoids
Colocynth	Colic
Colocynth	Diarrhoea
Colocynth	Sciatica
Croton tig	Nappy rash
Cucurbita pep	Morning sickness
Cuprum met	Cramp
Dioscorea	Colic
Drosera	Cough
Dulcamara	Rheumatic and arthritic pain
Equisetum	Bedwetting
Equisetum	Sleep problems
Eupatorium perf	Cold and flu
Euphrasia	Cold and flu
Euphrasia	Eye problems
Euphrasia	Hay fever
Ferrum phos	Abscesses and boils
Ferrum phos	Cold and flu
Ferrum phos	Fever
Ferrum phos	Nosebleed
Gelsemium	Anxiety and shock
Gelsemium	Cold and flu
Gelsemium	Cramp
Gelsemium	Fever
Gelsemium	Hay fever
Gelsemium	Sciatica
Gelsemium	Sore throat
Glonoine	Headache and migraine
Glonoine	Hot flushes
Gnaphalium	Sciatica
Graphites	Ear problems

Graphites	Eczema and dermatitis
Graphites	Eye problems
Graphites	Hot flushes
Gunpowder	Acne
Hamamelis	Bruising
Hamamelis	Haemorrhoids
Hamamelis	Menopause
Hamamelis	Nosebleed
Hepar sulph	Abscesses and boils
Hepar sulph	Acne
Hepar sulph	Catarrh and sinus problems
Hepar sulph	Cold sores
Hepar sulph	Cough
Hepar sulph	Ear problems
Hepar sulph	Sore throat
Hepar sulph	Wounds
Hydrastis	Catarrh and sinus problems
Hydrastis	Constipation
Hydrastis	Mouth problems
Hypericum	Backache
Hypericum	Bites and stings
Hypericum	Bruising
Hypericum	Chickenpox and shingles
Hypericum	Injury
Hypericum	Sports injuries
Hypericum	Wounds
Ignatia	Anxiety and shock
Ignatia	Headache and migraine
Ignatia	Menopause
Ipecac	Cough
Ipecac	Diarrhoea
Ipecac	Labour

Ipecac	Morning sickness
Ipecac	Nausea and vomiting
Iris vers	Headache and migraine
Jaborandi	Hot flushes
Kali bich	Catarrh and sinus problems
Kali brom	Acne
Kali carb	Backache
Kali iod	Catarrh and sinus problems
Kali mur	Ear problems
Kali phos	Fatigue (acute)
Kali phos	Labour
Kalmia	Chickenpox and shingles
Kalmia	Rheumatic and arthritic pain
Kreosotum	Mouth problems
Lac caninum	Breastfeeding
Lac caninum	Labour
Lac defloratum	Breastfeeding
Lac defloratum	Labour
Lachesis	Abscesses and boils
Lachesis	Bereavement
Lachesis	Catarrh and sinus problems
Lachesis	Headache and migraine
Lachesis	Hot flushes
Lachesis	Pre-menstrual syndrome
Ledum	Bites and stings
Ledum	Bruising
Ledum	Eye problems
Ledum	Gout
Ledum	Rheumatic and arthritic pain
Ledum	Sports injuries
Ledum	Wounds
Ledum tincture	Bites and stings

Lilium tig	Pre-menstrual syndrome
Lycopodium	Anxiety and shock
Lycopodium	Bedwetting
Lycopodium	Ear problems
Lycopodium	Flatulence
Lycopodium	Headache and migraine
Lycopodium	Perspiration
Lycopodium	Pre-menstrual syndrome
Lycopodium	Sciatica
Lycopodium	Urinary problems (acute)
Mag phos	Cramp
Mag phos	Period pains
Mag phos	Sciatica
Merc sol	Abscesses and boils
Merc sol	Cold and flu
Merc sol	Eye problems
Merc sol	Fatigue (acute)
Merc sol	Fever
Merc sol	Glandular fever
Merc sol	Mouth problems
Merc sol	Nappy rash
Merc sol	Perspiration
Merc sol	Sore throat
Merc sol	Teething
Mezereum	Catarrh and sinus problems
Mezereum	Chickenpox and shingles
Mezereum	Eczema and dermatitis
Millefolium	Nosebleed
Nat mur	Bereavement
Nat mur	Catarrh and sinus problems
Nat mur	Cold and flu
Nat mur	Cold sores

Nat mur	Headache and migraine
Nat mur	Itch
Nat mur	Pre-menstrual syndrome
Nat sulph	Sports injuries
Nux vom	Backache
Nux vom	Cold and flu
Nux vom	Colic
Nux vom	Constipation
Nux vom	Haemorrhoids
Nux vom	Headache and migraine
Nux vom	Morning sickness
Nux vom	Nausea and vomiting
Nux vom	Pre-menstrual syndrome
Nux vom	Sleep problems
Nux vom	Smoking
Nux vom	Teething
Nux vom	Urinary problems (acute)
Passiflora	Sleep problems
Petroleum	Eczema and dermatitis
Petroleum	Travel sickness
Phosphorus	Anxiety and shock
Phosphorus	Cough
Phosphorus	Mouth problems
Phosphorus	Nosebleed
Phosphorus	Sleep problems
Phosphorus	Sore throat
Phosphorus	Sports injuries
Phytolacca	Breastfeeding
Phytolacca	Sore throat
Plantago	Bedwetting
Plumbum met	Constipation
Podophyllum	Diarrhoea

Psorinum	Acne
Psorinum	Eczema and dermatitis
Pulsatilla	Bedwetting
Pulsatilla	Bereavement
Pulsatilla	Catarrh and sinus problems
Pulsatilla	Cough
Pulsatilla	Ear problems
Pulsatilla	Eye problems
Pulsatilla	Gout
Pulsatilla	Hot flushes
Pulsatilla	Menopause
Pulsatilla	Morning sickness
Pulsatilla	Nausea and vomiting
Pulsatilla	Nosebleed
Pulsatilla	Period pains
Pulsatilla	Pre-menstrual syndrome
Pyrogenium	Catarrh and sinus problems
Pyrogenium	Ear problems
Ranunc bulb	Chickenpox and shingles
Raphanus	Flatulence
Rhododendron	Rheumatic and arthritic pain
Rhus tox	Acne
Rhus tox	Backache
Rhus tox	Chickenpox and shingles
Rhus tox	Cold and flu
Rhus tox	Cold sores
Rhus tox	Cramp
Rhus tox	Eczema and dermatitis
Rhus tox	Gout
Rhus tox	Itch
Rhus tox	Nappy rash
Rhus tox	Rheumatic and arthritic pain

Rhus tox	Sciatica
Rhus tox	Sprains and strains
Ruta grav	Backache
Ruta grav	Bruising
Ruta grav	Sprains and strains
Sabadilla	Eye problems
Sabadilla	Hay fever
Sabal serr	Urinary problems (acute)
Sabina	Warts and verrucae
Sanguinaria	Acne
Sanguinaria	Headache and migraine
Sarsaparilla	Urinary problems (acute)
Scutellaria	Fatigue (acute)
Sempervivum	Cold sores
Sepia	Bereavement
Sepia	Hot flushes
Sepia	Morning sickness
Sepia	Period pains
Sepia	Pre-menstrual syndrome
Silica	Abscesses and boils
Silica	Acne
Silica	Breastfeeding
Silica	Constipation
Silica	Headache and migraine
Silica	Mouth problems
Silica	Perspiration
Silica	Urinary problems (acute)
Silica	Wounds
Sol	Burns
Sol	Itch
Spigelia	Chickenpox and shingles
Spigelia	Headache and migraine

Spongia	Cough
Stannum met	Cough
Staphisagria	Breastfeeding
Staphisagria	Eye problems
Staphisagria	Headache and migraine
Staphisagria	Smoking
Staphisagria	Urinary problems (acute)
Sticta	Catarrh and sinus problems
Sulphur	Acne
Sulphur	Constipation
Sulphur	Diarrhoea
Sulphur	Eczema and dermatitis
Sulphur	Hot flushes
Sulphur	Nappy rash
Sulphur	Perspiration
Sulphur iodatum	Acne
Symphoricarpus	Morning sickness
Symphytum	Bruising
Symphytum	Eye problems
Symphytum	Injury
Symphytum	Sports injuries
Tabacum	Travel sickness
Thuja	Headache and migraine
Thuja	Warts and verrucae
Tuberculinum bovinum (Tub bov)	Coughs
Urtica	Bites and stings
Urtica	Burns
Urtica	Gout
Urtica	Itch
Verat alb	Cramp
Verat alb	Diarrhoea
Zinc met	Cramp
Zinc met	Fatigue (acute)

Index

Entries in *italics* indicate ailments listed in the prescribing charts.